To my family
and the memory of
Sarai Ribicoff

Acknowledgments

Even if he prefers Coke to coffee, William Whitworth, the editor emeritus of *The Atlantic Monthly,* generously commissioned the series of four articles that led to this book and allowed me the freedom to write it. Cullen Murphy edited the articles, with Martha Spaulding and Barbara Wallraff; Eric Haas, Leonie Foy and Sue Parilla checked the facts. More important even than the invaluable improvements they made were the patience and good humor they and everyone else at *The Atlantic* showed while I worked on this book. It can only be described as wondrous, and I cannot imagine a better family of colleagues.

For the original series of articles, Tim Castle led me to many rich sources of information and was one himself. For both the articles and the book, George Howell let me use the headquarters of The Coffee Connection, in Boston, as library and laboratory, and he gave unstintingly of his great expertise and critical skill. Robert Dattala also spent many hours educating me, and Ray Trevino, Jordan Wood and others then at The Coffee Connection helped shepherd me through the puzzles of buying, roasting and packaging coffee.

I received the unexpected and invaluable gift of the expert reading of these chapters from Jerry Baldwin, of Peet's Coffee, in the Bay Area; Kevin M. Knox, formerly of Allegro Coffee Company, in Thornton, Colorado; Bruce E. Mullins, of Coffee Bean International, in Portland; and Donald N. Schoenholt, of Gillies Coffee, in Brooklyn. These men gave extraordinary time and attention to pointing out my many errors of fact and their many disagreements over taste. In reading and rereading their extensive comments, I forged my own opinions and knowledge. They and George Howell are my masters. The book is immeasurably strengthened for their corrections and guidance; any errors are mine.

Other early educators include Alfred Peet, the founder of the California shops that helped launch America's interest in quality coffee; Phyllis Baldenhofer, now of the George Alexander House, in Healdsburg, California; Daniel C. Cox, now of Coffee Enterprises, in Burlington, Vermont; Alf Kramer, at the Nordic Coffee Center; Tim McCormack, at Caravali Coffees, in Seattle;

The Joy of Coffee

The Joy of Coffee

The Essential Guide to Buying, Brewing and Enjoying

Revised and Updated

Corby Kummer

Photographs by Jim Scherer
Illustrations by Evangelia Philippidis

Houghton Mifflin Company
Boston · New York

Library of Congress Cataloging-in-Publication Data

Kummer, Corby

The joy of coffee: the essential guide to buying, brewing and
enjoying / Corby Kummer ; photographs by Jim Scherer;
illustrations by Evangelia Philippidis. — Rev. and updated

p. cm

Includes bibliographical references and index.

ISBN 0-618-30240-9

1. Coffee brewing 2. Coffee 3. Cookery (Coffee) I. Title.

TX817.C6K86 2003

641.8'77 — dc21   2003047877

Printed and bound in the United States of America

QUM 10 9 8 7 6 5 4 3

Design by Elizabeth Johnsboen

Barbara Westfield and Ike Komatsu, at Salton. Ian Bersten remained a long-time, irrepressible source of information.

I invaded the London headquarters of the International Coffee Organization, and my incessant questioning was graciously tolerated by Katharine Winchester, Mary Banks, Alejandro Feria Morales and Pedro Kari. Andrea Ditta, at the Biblioteca Internazionale La Vigna, in Vicenza, Italy, pointed me toward many sources on coffee, as did Daniela Ball and Barbara Blumer, of the Jacobs Suchard Museum in Zurich.

Dave Olsen showed me many unexpected pleasures of espresso at the gleaming Starbucks headquarters, then freshly built, in Seattle, and he, Howard Schultz and Mary Williams continued to be generous with help and expertise. Mary Williams, an intrepid hunter of beans, was especially informative about how coffees vary by where they are grown.

Bill McAlpin was both an extremely generous host and an exacting one, wanting visitors to know just why the people who raise coffee make so much difference to the way it tastes. Green Mountain Coffee Roasters made possible my visit to La Minita, McAlpin's Costa Rican plantation, and at Green Mountain, Paul Comey, Bob Stiller and Susan Williams marshaled expert opinions on various topics. While I was in Costa Rica, Carole Kurtz and Carter Vincent also made my stay the inspiration it was. Sven Dahler, of Bernhard Rothfos AG, in Hamburg, introduced me to the fast-paced world of a coffee brokerage.

In my various espresso-searching excursions in Italy, the Illy clan, led by Dr. Ernesto Illy and his sons, Riccardo (lately mayor of Trieste), Francesco and Andrea were unfailingly hospitable and ready with explanations and on-site visits; Denise Tecchio coordinated everything, and Sergio Michel and Marino Petracco patiently led me through technical questions. In Scottsdale, Arizona, Alain Rastrelly showed me Illy's American side.

On the other side of the country, at Lavazza, in Turin, Ennio Ranaboldo, Daniela Arneodo and Giuseppe Lavazza gave me similar welcome and assistance; and in Lavazza's New York office, Alberto Paderi, Elizabeth Kane and Mitchel Margulis provided many kinds of help, though they were often given no advance warning. In Florence, Piero Bambi, at La Marzocco, in the hills of Florence, taught me much about the innards of espresso machines; Mario Muttoni, of Spidem, explained the technology of filter holders. Piero Busolini showed me his family espresso roaster, Udinese Caffe, in Udine.

In America, I learned much about espresso from Kent Bakke at Espresso Specialists, in Seattle; Mark Bishop, at Espresso Northeast, in Rhode Island; Umberto Bizzarri and David Baron, at Torrefazione Italia, in Seattle; Mauro R. Cipolla, at Caffé D'arte, in Seattle; Carlo Middione, at Vivande Porta Via, in San Francisco; Carlo di Ruocco, at Mr. Espresso, in Oakland; Bernard N. Mariano, at Xcell, in Chicago; Mark Mooradian, at Espresso Express, in the Boston area; Tim O'Connor, at Pacific Espresso, in Santa Cruz; and David C. Schomer, a barista's barista, at Espresso Vivace, in Seattle.

Any work of nonfiction stands on its accuracy, as the fact checkers at *The Atlantic* have taught me—and so I prevailed upon a number of them to help check this book. Katie Bacon, Gina Hahn, Julia Parker and Jane Rosenzweig jokingly called themselves "Corby's Angels," but angelic they truly were. Without them, I could never have finished.

For expert reading of the caffeine chapter, I thank Roland R. Griffiths, of Johns Hopkins University Medical School, and Eric Rimm, of the Harvard School of Public Health; for help in understanding caffeine, Richard Greenberg, of the Institute of Food Technologists, and Richard Wurtman, of the Massachusetts Institute of Technology; and for help with decaffeination, Peter Frey, at Kaffee Veredelungs Werk, in Hamburg, Don G. McDonald, of Jacobs Suchard Canada, Marc Sims, of the American Natural Decaf Company, in Berkeley, and Thomas Mühlnikel, Rudolf Zobel and Pasquale Peluso, of the SDD decaffeination plant near Venafro, Italy.

Charles Mann lent an expert writer's and editor's eye to many drafts. Michael Sivetz brought his lifetime of expertise to looking at several chapters, but his always vigorous disagreements mean that no book but his own will have his imprimatur; I am grateful for his attention and clarification.

I was also set right by Ted R. Lingle, head of the Specialty Coffee Association of America, where Melissa J. Pugash was helpful. Erna Knutsen, another revered figure in the coffee trade, was generous with her expertise on coffee cultivation and processing. Charles Bosworth, of Dallis Brothers, in New York, gave information on water, that crucial element in brewing. Lilian Cheung, Jessica Mitford, Paul Rozin, Jeffrey Steingarten and Paula Wolfert generously supplied various references.

Lisë Stern, an exceptionally talented baker and candymaker, developed most of the recipes for this book, sharing her own long-practiced treasures and patiently baking batch after batch of the cookies and cakes that existed only in my hungry imagination. Friends don't come any better than Flo Braker. She rounded out the recipe collection with favorites from her private trove. Jim Scherer, a stellar Boston photographer, brought his usual precision and elegance to showing the coffee equipment—and a genuine enthusiasm for coffee too.

With his brisk humor, Rafe Sagalyn is an ideal agent. Harriet Bell helped me conceive of the book, and Ann Bramson offered advice. Editors and friends who helped me to survive and to stay interested in coffee include Kurt Andersen, Amy Gross, Isolde Motley, Nancy Moore, Maggie Simmons, Margot Slade, Nancy Smith and Susan Wyland.

Pam Hunter and Carl Doumani's writers' colony was serenely perfect. Leonardo Tondo similarly provided shelter in a beautiful place and gave a discerning layman's reading too. Understanding friends weathered lapsed communication and checked in to ask about the book—or whether they shouldn't ask: Keith Alexander, David Berreby, William Castronuovo, Francis Davis, Mark Furstenberg, Seymour and Elizabeth Hersh, Margo Howard, Kate Jakobsen, Sheryl Julian, Ellen Kennelly, Michael Kimmelman, Sarah Lowengard, M. G. Lord, Patricia Marx, Lawrence F. O'Donnell, Jr., Peggy Pierrepont, Erika Pilver, Jennifer Quale, the Rosenbloom family, Sandra Shapiro, Lisa Wagner and Dorothy Zinberg were among the kindhearted. Ken Mayer gave loving support when it was most needed.

My life has been greatly enriched by La Banda, an informal group of writers and friends who, when not traveling together in Italy, dream that they are—and try to finish books: Ed Behr, Carol Field, Nancy Harmon Jenkins, Fred Plotkin and Faith Heller Willinger. Dun Gifford, Greg Drescher and Sara Baer-Sinnott at Oldways enabled me to pursue coffee in exotic locations I could never otherwise have visited. Tony May and the Gruppo Ristoratori Italiani and, at the Italian Trade Commission, Giorgio Lulli, Augusto Marchini, Hermelina Ressa and Morley Timons helped me revisit espresso's homeland; Maria Bergamin, Julia Buonocore, Clara Chernin, Marta-Marie Lotti and Rosa-maria Zannino Grippa at Alitalia helped smooth the kinks of travel.

A fellow writer who had his choice of publishers, Richard Sax, told me that he chose Chapters Books so that he would be proud to have his name on the book. Every writer lucky enough to work with Rux Martin shares his feelings. I came to understand that the rare moments when I was satisfied with a chapter would elicit soonest her gentle preface, "I have just a few questions," which would lead to my rewriting every single paragraph—a process that was frequently repeated. She was always right, and I'll always be grateful. Alice Lawrence is an infinitely patient and reassuring copy editor, and Barry Estabrook a deus ex machina.

Rux championed this updating and revision in her current celebrated reign at Houghton Mifflin, and I'm grateful to Houghton for keeping alive such an important part of my life. John Auerbach inspired me, as in so much else, to pay caring attention to the people who grow coffee. Without the fantastically thorough, persistent and able help of Ben Healy, this new edition would have been inconceivable.

The impetus for this book came from Barbara Kafka, a friend of rare substance and sustenance who is challenging and loving in equal measure. The original series of *Atlantic Monthly* articles was written one August in the farmhouse she shares with her husband, Ernest, and her married children, Nicole, Richard, Michael and Jill. A few years later, on another August day in the same house, as she watched me go through yet another carton of research materials, she said, "There's a time when you have to stop reading and start writing." I went upstairs and began.

Contents

Preface to the 2003 Edition

In the twenty years since I began obsessively researching coffee, it has become a lot easier to find a good cup in the United States. Where I live, in Boston, I have American coffee history and the always changing world of beans from distant lands within easy reach. I can drink the benchmark blends of Peet's, the Berkeley-based chain that inspired the American movement for coffee with real flavor and integrity, and buy the beans to brew my own at home. I frequent cafés that use beans roasted in Seattle by Batdorf & Bronson or Torrefazione Italia, two companies that rode the quality-coffee wave and managed to keep afloat after it crested. I can stop in for a cup of defining East Coast coffee at Dunkin' Donuts, the ubiquitous chain that got its start near Boston and has been influenced by the national move toward better beans. If I want to buy extremely fresh roasted beans, I can watch the process through a neat plastic window at a gleaming new branch of Whole Foods, the national chain of supermarkets dedicated to raising the standards of how food is raised and sold. A few years ago, Whole Foods bought a pioneering Colorado coffee roaster, Allegro, and incorporated its mission to educate people and supply fine beans. Or I can go to the gleaming new Copacafé, the brainchild of one of America's coffee greats, George Howell, who is roasting just a few of the world's finest coffees, hoping to bring world attention—and higher prices—to the people who grow them.

All these companies show America's increased focus on coffee quality, which is probably unrivaled in any other country except Japan or Italy. They also show the reality of how the coffee renaissance, which was steaming through the country just when the first edition of this book appeared, has shaken out. What I can no longer do is go from alternative café to café, where impassioned hobbyists turned semi-professional fuss over roasting machines that look like old locomotives and waft heavenly smells through the store and the neighborhood.

This is because of Starbucks, the Goliath of the coffee world. From the time I began chronicling coffee, I have watched Starbucks move from a company with ambitions to increase its Seattle base a bit north and south to a national chain that bought out and dissolved many competitors—including, most notably, The Coffee Connection, a Boston-based beacon of quality for the whole country which was founded by Howell. Now, of course, Starbucks is an international company practically as famous as McDonald's—and a similarly reviled and admired symbol of America.

Starbucks changed our view and expectations of coffee. Whatever can be said about its expansion techniques and the commodification of the quirky delights of café life, the company has made an immense number of people care about decent coffee and allowed them to find and drink it. Critics point out that Starbucks plowed over the independent local competition in its drive for hegemony. I, too, miss the many small, dedicated experimental roasters who proudly display prize burlap coffee sacks on the wall and urge customers to try their latest find. Such impassioned people are the transmitters of coffee wisdom—the people who can set others on lifelong quests to find, as The Coffee Connection's slogan had it, "the ultimate cup."

Expert coffee men like George Howell, Jerry Baldwin and Ernesto Illy gave me my education—and will give you yours, in the pages of this book. While the independent, dreaming roasters will always have my heart, it is Starbucks that holds the key to the future. The origin of the company was an idealistic group of men, including Baldwin, who wanted people to sample and enjoy the coffee they discovered and loved. The degree of personalization changed utterly as the approach became sheerly corporate. This everyone knows. There's plenty more to criticize, too, about Starbucks, including the varying degree of freshness in beans roasted thousands of miles away and the dark roasts that can smudge the delicate differences coffee farmers sweat and sacrifice to achieve.

But it is also true that thanks to Starbucks, a wealth of coffee information and, yes, coffee quality is available to millions more people than a few years ago. Starbucks held the line at flavored coffees, which as the coffee fad took hold threatened to paint the country in lurid crayon colors, and bought a leading espresso-machine maker to provide the shiny, steaming heart of its stores.

And then there's the crucial question of the welfare of coffee farmers and the land they work—the question that has become foremost to anyone who loves coffee and cares about the world, the question that has taken on urgency since the first edition of this book appeared. Here, too, Starbucks holds the key. With its worldwide reach and immense buying power, Starbucks has the ability to affect the future of coffee with the choices it makes and the policies it sets.

Especially in the last few years, the outlook for quality coffee hasn't been good. Fewer and fewer farmers can make a living. The news in recent years has been the startling rise of Vietnam from a very minor producer to the world's second largest, after Brazil—heartening for a Southeast Asian country with a tormented history but terrible for Central and South America, home to relatively disorganized groups of smallholders who have the potential to grow great coffee. So do farmers in many parts of sub-Saharan Africa, which, since the book came out, has only become more politically troubled, meaning that distribution is uncertain even when good beans are grown and processed. Both Latin America and Africa have the altitude and cool nights required for arabica, the species of coffee with real flavor. All coffee in Vietnam is robusta, the low-growing kind that can withstand the heat and humidity of Southeast Asia. Robusta is cheap filler coffee.

The bright spots in the business today are the increasing number and ambition of groups that aim to help small farmers. The International Coffee Organization, for decades the cartel that attempted to keep prices reasonable by having its members stockpile coffee, has for the first time since the 1980s announced the revival of a price agreement. This could be good news for many member farmers, who for years have been forced to sell their crops at a loss. The ICO is also trying to improve the quality of coffee in its member countries—overdue efforts by a long-moribund group.

When I first wrote this book, people were coming alive to the idea that coffee could have real taste and realizing that something they'd viewed as simply a commodity that woke them up in the morning could have a wonderful range of flavors, flavors anyone could capture at home. Now coffee drinkers are awakening to the recognition that it is *people* who grow the beans, that families work to raise coffee trees, and that their labor and sometimes love should always be amply rewarded.

As in agriculture everywhere, though, middlemen pocket payments that rightfully belong to the farmer. Several groups that existed when I wrote the book have expanded their programs in the hopes of righting this wrong. Equal Exchange, a for-profit and right-minded group, pioneered the concept in the United States of buying and selling organic Fair Trade coffee from farmers and cooperatives in Latin America, Asia and Africa. The international Fair Trade program requires importers to guarantee farmers a minimum price and extend credit to them, and it provides technical assistance to help farmers make the transition to organic growing. Oxfam, the international aid group, has taken an active interest in coffee growers, devising a Coffee Rescue Plan to encourage big international companies to buy more Fair Trade coffee. Paying the modestly higher price for Fair Trade beans will make an enormous difference to the future of farmers around the world as well as the future of the environment— a concept Oxfam hopes roasters large and small will understand. Part of the plan requires large growers to destroy stocks of coffee that do not meet the International Coffee Organization's minimum quality standards, thus giving small farmers a better chance to sell all their coffee at a decent price. Coffee Kids takes a different approach, enlisting coffee merchants and individual consumers to contribute money that it redirects to community development and education and health programs. This directly improves the lives and futures of farmers and their families—even if those futures mean livelihoods not involved with the difficult practice of farming coffee.

George Howell, ever the visionary, thinks that the only solution for farmers and drinkers who care about quality is to establish an identity for individual farmers. After he sold The Coffee Connection, he worked for several years in Brazil and Central America to establish the Cup of Excellence, a rigorous tasting competition that brings small farmers to the attention of buyers around the world—and, through an Internet auction of their tiny but fantastic annual crop, brings the winners rich rewards and, crucially, name recognition.

Since the first edition of this book, the interest in organic and sustainable agriculture coffee has increased. Shade-grown coffee is less economically efficient than coffee grown with no taller trees to shelter it. But it tastes much better, because the longer growing cycle means the possibility of greater flavor. Shade-grown coffee is also immeasurably better for the survival of other kinds of crops and birds and wildlife than beans grown on land stripped of shade trees—for years the standard way to grow coffee.

People who care about flavor and quality ask whether any of these groups—however laudable and essential they are to the future of small farmers and the environment—actually help the cause of better-tasting coffee. The answer is that some do and many do not. Their priorities are the welfare of the growers far more than the preference of the consumer. Unless farmers pay closer attention to planting practices and especially to better processing and storage, countries that produce huge amounts of mediocre beans will continue to force small farmers with the potential of producing great (or at least good) coffee out of business.

No matter how lovingly raised, of course, nothing can rescue badly made coffee. Here's where *The Joy of Coffee* can change your life. I had fun puzzling out the rules of brewing in various machines and have been extremely gratified to see, on various websites, my experimental formulations carry the weight of stone-etched commandments. Since the book came out, there has been no great leap forward in brewing machines or methods. The small changes here and there are noted in the completely updated Sources.

Coffee is a blessing and a gift. A well-made cup gets close to heaven. The making part is easy, and there are dozens of tips in this book that even followed one at a time can radically improve the quality of the coffee you make at home. As for the beans, I'll just say as a last word that I hope you seek out a roaster who cares about where every bean came from and who does something, however small, to help the people who raise them. Big ideas start small, and helping small farmers grow better beans is a big idea in which every coffee drinker can take part.

— C.K.
January 2003

The Joy
of Coffee

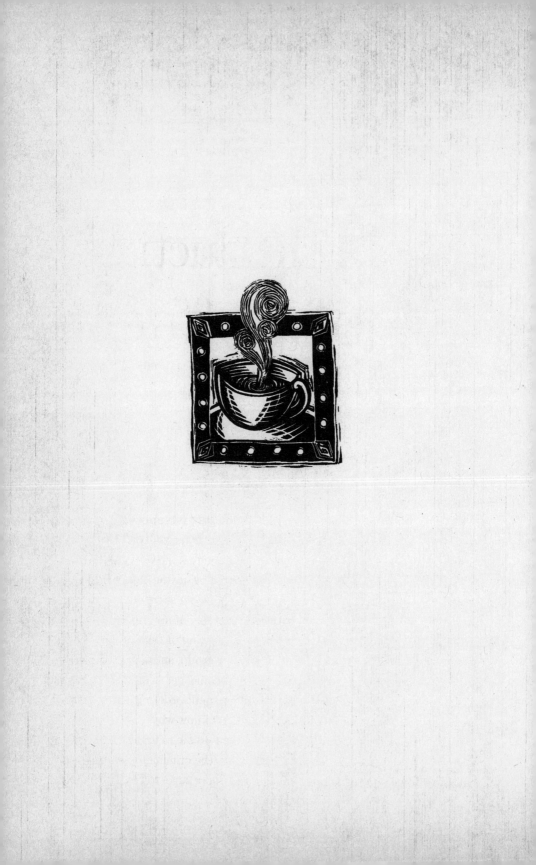

Introduction

M Y COFFEE EDUCATION BEGAN at full speed when I tried to keep up with the instructions and opinions coming at me from a group of coffee experts—fanatics, really. Wanting to write about coffee in the mid-1980s, I had come to San Francisco to hang out at espresso bars, which at the time were hard to find. On the very first day of my trip, someone told me I was in luck: just then was the annual meeting of the Specialty Coffee Association of America, a small and fairly new group, and if I wangled an invitation to its opening cocktail reception, I could get a jump-start on my research. I thought my time would be better spent ordering espresso, but I went anyway. I knew I loved coffee. I just didn't know why.

Faster than my pen could write, people told me in urgent bursts about the superiority of arabica beans over robustas, the criminally destructive hot plates on home and restaurant brewers, the importance to the true connoisseur of single-estate coffees. Seemingly everyone in the room gathered around me, talking over each other as if this were the one chance they'd get to convey everything they had learned. Even though I don't drink coffee at night, a cup suddenly seemed like a good idea.

Finally, the owner of a local specialty-coffee shop, who had silenced everyone else to deliver a long monologue about when to cut off the airflow in a drum roaster, stopped herself. "You have to understand," she said by way of apology. "We all love the bean."

Over the next eight years, while standing behind espresso-bar counters, beside huge industrial roasters and in rooms where professionals taste hundreds of cups a day to evaluate beans, I learned to understand and even speak the language sprayed at me that first night. I had a wonderful, long trip researching coffee up and down Italy, across America and even in South America and Germany, meeting people everywhere who had spent their lives passionately devoted to the bean.

Throughout my journey, I kept looking for better and better answers to the basic questions I began with: What matters most in buying coffee? How can you sort through the jumble of place names and whimsical labels on beans and blends? Is a dark roast better, more sophisticated, than a light roast? Is it essential to grind coffee beans at home? How can you keep coffee fresh after you buy it? What are the best brewing methods, and do you have to buy a new machine to try them? How do you pick and use the right equipment? How is espresso different from brewed coffee? How can you make densely flavored, silkily foamy cappuccinos and caffè lattes at home?

I also wondered just how bad for you caffeine can be, because I wouldn't want to go a day without coffee, and every year there seems to be a new verdict. I sifted through hundreds of articles and found that although caffeine probably won't take any time off your life, dependence on it to get you through the day carries its own price. Because everyone's sensitivity to caffeine is different, and my own sensitivity is high, I searched out the newest methods of decaffeination, hoping to find coffee with more body and flavor than the rinse water I was used to.

I found it, and much more. In back rooms of warehouses, in bean-filled holding rooms on German docks, in decaffeination plants in southern Italy, in shrines to espresso in Rome and Naples and in dozens of the new coffeehouses that opened all across America while I continued my search, I learned some fundamental truths about coffee: Freshness matters more than just about anything. Nothing is as sophisticated as your own taste buds. No kind of coffee will keep for very long, and the freezer is by no means a better storage choice than a countertop or cupboard.

I learned, too, that a few very simple steps can drastically improve your everyday brew. Using metal filters instead of paper, for instance, or letting boiled water cool for a few seconds before pouring it over ground coffee, or just making sure you clean the brewer thoroughly every so often—little tricks make gigantic differences.

No one bean is best. Once you know some of the main differences, you have to decide what pleases you the most in a cup of coffee. Before you know what your favorite bean or blend is, you should put yourself in the hands of someone like the woman at that San Francisco conference who tastes dozens of coffee samples a month before selecting the beans she will roast in her own store. If you don't have someone like that where you live, it's easy to find such a person at the other end of the phone who will mail you fresh-roasted beans.

After talking to every expert I could find—and sipping more cups of delicious coffee than I imagined existed—I collected a mountain of information and tips. This book contains the best of what I learned: enough to help you have much, much better coffee than you're used to and to appreciate the whole culture that has grown up around coffee. The group that met in such small, clubby quarters in San Francisco has grown explosively; that hotel room wouldn't hold even one of its subcommittees today.

In these chapters, I'll take you through a coffee plantation, where, midway through my research, I became reinspired by the smell of coffee blossoms and the sight of fruit-bearing coffee trees on volcanic Costa Rican hillsides. I'll take you into the mills, where the beans are liberated from the fruits, dried and raked on big patios and carefully prepared for shipping; and into secretive "cupping rooms," where experts who sip and spit dozens of samples a day decide which beans you'll find in a supermarket can or in a bag at a fancy coffee shop. We'll visit the noisy floors of roasting plants, where men and women with the skill and sensitivity of chefs decide how to unlock the flavors in each kind of bean.

Finally, I'll take you into your own kitchen, where I'll show you exactly how to make coffee as wonderful as the cup you remember from a vacation long ago—the one that tasted better than all the cups since. Because I enjoy a cup of really good coffee even more with a delicious cookie or piece of cake beside it, the last chapter is devoted to mostly sweet, and a few not-so-sweet, things that make coffee taste better, and certainly make drinking it more fun. At the end are sources for the equipment and coffee beans I recommend.

The point of my long journey was never to become a coffee insider. It was to enhance the pleasure I take in something that I will probably drink every day for the rest of my life. I hope to enhance your daily pleasure too.

Growing Beans

1

SIPPING A FROTHY CAPPUCCINO or a "regular" with cream and sugar, it can be hard to remember that coffee is the seed of a fruit that grows on trees. Like any fruit, it tastes of where it grew: of the soil, be it volcanic and loamy or crumbly red clay; of the tempestuous summer rains that clear by evening; of the high, hot morning sun and the cool night winds of the dry season.

Connoisseurs will forever argue over just what makes a coffee great. But most people familiar with the art of raising coffee agree that among the best-run coffee plantations in the world is La Minita, in the mountains of Costa Rica. The coffee that bears its name is one of the increasingly available "single-estate" coffees, meaning beans grown on just one farm rather than a blend from many farms and many countries. It is on anyone's short list of the world's finest. The immense care that is taken at La Minita, from enriching the soil to hand-picking the fruits of the coffee tree to processing the beans inside the fruit, illustrates why coffee tastes so different depending not only on where it grows but also on who grows it.

When I paid a January visit to La Minita, toward the end of the bustling, sprawling, cheerful activity of a coffee harvest, I finally found the missing link in my long apprenticeship as an unprofessional coffee taster. I thought I knew a lot about tasting coffee. Going where I had never been, though—to a place where coffee grows—reinspired me. Seeing the passion and work that went into growing the commodity I had encountered only in big burlap sacks or little plastic sample bags made me fall in love with coffee all over again. I also made an idiot of myself, trying to learn to be a coffee picker.

The Gospel of Arabica

The list of the world's best coffee almost invariably includes beans from Guatemala and Costa Rica in Central America and, going far back to the origins of cultivated coffee, Ethiopia, Yemen and Kenya. These countries have something in common: an equatorial location and a mountainous subtropical climate, which produces the most fragrant and intensely flavored beans. Fine coffee is *Coffea arabica* (a-*rab*-ica), named for its original popularizers, the Arabs, who brought it from its native East Africa to the Arabian Peninsula in the fifteenth century. All the delicate, prized flavors possible in coffee are found in arabica. The new shops that offer freshly roasted beans are putting arabica beans, not robusta, into their machines.

Arabica beans don't do well in very hot and humid weather, flourishing instead in places that offer warm but not fierce days and chilly nights, with temperatures often as low as the fifties but not much lower, and an extended rainy season. Extreme cold is a mortal enemy of any kind of coffee plant. Frosts kill coffee trees, freezing the sap and rupturing their tissues. The greatest disruption to coffee production in this century was a terrible freeze in Brazil in 1975, skyrocketing prices. Disputes over stockpiling among coffee-raising countries further disrupted the market, sending prices so far down that many farmers had to sell their plantations. Just the threat of a frost in 1997 unsettled the market for months.

The finickiness of arabica beans and the labor problems of farming at three thousand to six thousand feet (think of getting your footing on mountainsides day in and day out) mean it's small wonder that the other commercially important coffee species—robusta, or *Coffea canephora*— caught on fast. Robusta grows very well at sea level, requiring little more than a tropical or semitropical climate. Native to West rather than East Africa, robust a shares none of the exalted history of arabica. It was first cultivated widely a mere hundred years ago for its low cost and hardiness. It shares none of arabica's exalted taste either. The chief flavor attribute of robusta, which dominates just about any blend you buy in a can, is that of a brown paper bag.

Some longtime coffee observers think that the reason "specialty coffee" has seen such explosive growth in the past few years after a thirty-year decline in American coffee consumption is that big commercial coffee companies—the ones that put cans onto supermarket shelves—fell asleep. Colas muscled in on coffee as America's preferred caffeine-delivery system, because coffee packers started putting higher and higher ratios of robusta beans into their blends, driving down both price and quality and sending consumers to the soda aisle. Finally, in the late 1960s, a few people who cared about coffee rediscovered and reintroduced coffee with real flavor—arabica coffee. The gospel spread slowly in the 1970s and finally won large numbers of converts in the late 1980s, setting the stage for the flood of coffee bars of the 1990s. For those interested in watching their caffeine consumption, arabica offers a crucial advantage besides having infinitely greater flavor than robusta: it has about half the caffeine.

A Model Plantation

La Minita is a showplace of raising and processing coffee because of the passion of its owner, Bill McAlpin. McAlpin is an oversized man in his fifties who grew up in a family whose agricultural holdings included a large coffee plantation along the Fila de Bustamonte range of central Costa Rica, a ninety-minute drive south of the capital, San José. In 1976, he took over the family coffee farms, and through the early 1980s, he sold off land where the wind was too strong or the exposure to the sun less than ideal, all the while improving the heart of the farm.

The road from San José, much of it rocky and rutted, winds up and up the five thousand feet to La Minita, passing through blue-green mountains as spectacular as the Andes. Along most of them, coffee trees are planted on very steep slopes. It seems incredible that anyone could tend, let alone pick, these trees. Above seven thousand feet in Costa Rica, coffee won't grow. At those altitudes, visible in the distance, the landscape changes to grass-covered peaks with lines of trees like a checkerboard drawn by a child, denoting property lines for cattle pastures. On either side of the road, hibiscus, bougainvillea, impatiens and other blatantly colored wildflowers grow—an echo of the unchecked growth in the hundreds of square miles of the country's protected rain forests.

The deep green, leafy coffee plants that line the hillsides are kept so short that they look more like bushes than trees. The only recognizable trees are shade trees, either banana or other varieties, planted in a big grid. Shade trees protect coffee by helping to diffuse overzealous sunlight during the day and by keeping the air relatively warm at night. The bushlike height of the coffee trees—rarely more than five feet—makes them easier to pick. A few plantations still let their coffee plants grow beyond eight feet, the usual maximum height for arabica. Unrestricted trees can reach up to thirty feet, but these heights require workers to get up on ladders, meaning a loss of time and possible damage to the trees—workers must bend branches to reach the fruit. Most farms, like La Minita, cut back their trees to maintain a convenient height. The trees on La Minita are young, too—never more than fifteen years old, at which point they have lost much of their vigor and are dug up and replaced. It is rare to find productive trees more than twenty-five years old.

The land at La Minita is covered with fresh, impeccably tended trees of a cultivar called Caturra, which sixty years ago did not even exist. The truism is that old varieties—what farmers call heirlooms—produce coffee with the best, winiest flavor. This is a matter of controversy. Choosing the right variety certainly matters greatly to flavor, but so do soil and climate. A hallowed old variety like Bourbon—the basis of Latin American trade for hundreds of years—is an impractical choice for a farmer today, because its yield is one-third to one-half that of many new arabica varieties. The only place to find an heirloom variety is on an old farm whose owners could not afford to buy new trees or on a modern one whose owners are able to charge a premium for beans from old varieties.

Most experts who have tasted old varieties against new ones bred for production and hardiness report that the flavor of the older ones is more nuanced. It's a comparison few specialty merchants or their customers can make for themselves, because samples sent by brokers are identified by place of origin and date of harvest but rarely by variety. (A broker should immediately say if a sample is arabica or robusta, but sometimes even this is left vague.) Too, for a comparison to be fair, the old and new bean varieties should have been raised in the same soil and the same climate.

A greater threat to the future of high-quality coffee than new varieties of arabica may be breeds incorporating both arabica and robusta. Even if robusta has a dead flavor, it is nonetheless valuable to farmers for its resistance to various blights. Such hybrids are already being raised on a large scale in some South American countries, and breeding experiments are taking place in Kenya, where arabicas that coffee tasters revere grow on hillsides at fifty-five hundred to seven thousand feet. These efforts distress coffee lovers, even if Kenyans understandably want to protect their plants against Coffee Berry Disease—a fungus that is dangerously difficult to control.

Fungicides are relatively gentle: mostly based on copper, they pose a danger neither to the environment nor to the health of the people who apply them. The same is not true of herbicides and pesticides, which do harm workers, although probably not coffee drinkers—they are said not to penetrate to the coffee beans within the fruits of the tree, and certainly not to appear in brewed coffee in any dangerous quantity. The tradeoff facing farmers and connoisseurs the world over is delicate flavor versus disease resistance.

Painstaking Harvest

La Minita may not have the primeval beauty of Kenyan plantations that spread across plains and follow softly rolling hills on a high, high basin, or the drama of the volcanic cones all around the Guatemalan city of Antigua. But it is stunning nonetheless. Its verdant sugarloafs jut right into the sky—they are cloud-high. I visited La Minita toward the end of the harvest, which takes place between November and February. The plantation is in a region with just one rainy and one dry season, so there is only one harvest. In other climates, including coastal regions of Costa Rica, there can be as many as four or five harvests a year. The longer the ripening time and the cooler the air, the more time the beans will have to develop flavor. The most intensely flavored beans grow at high altitudes in places with a single harvest.

At La Minita, I finally understood why the range of flavors in coffee is described in terms used for fruits. Coffee beans are the seeds of a berry, called a "cherry" for the shape and for the deep crimson color of a fully ripe fruit. The even, ovoid shape resembles more a holly berry or plump cranberry.

I arrived at the plantation during the peak of activity, and McAlpin made me enter into it practically without giving me time to drop my bags. He presented me with a rattan basket and a long cord with a pad to attach it to my waist, and set me to picking. None of the terrain is level, and although I had been pointed to one of the flattest areas on the seven hundred acres, standing in one place was no easy trick. Slung around my waist, the big basket—about 16 inches in diameter and a foot deep—blocked my view of the ground. The crumbly clay soil didn't make things easier.

Neither did the vegetation growing between the trees. Plants between trees prevent soil erosion. Controlling rather than killing weeds—the approach adopted by organic farmers in many parts of the world, and the approach McAlpin takes—costs much more money than the blanket application of herbicides. Three times a year, workers with machetes shaped like scimitars rotate around La Minita, cutting back weeds. Shade trees are heavily pruned at the beginning of the rainy season, when the sun must reach the coffee plants to effect photosynthesis; sunlight also discourages fungal diseases. During the dry season, shade trees are instead allowed to luxuriate, because sunlight can burn coffee tree leaves.

The distribution of fruit on a coffee tree varies annoyingly. Twiglike branches splay out from the central trunk, which is usually no more than an inch or two in diameter. Most often, cherries cluster all along them, so a picker can position a basket just beneath and pull off the fruit. But cherries hide, too, in clusters or in ones and twos, often near the top and sometimes under leaves close to the ground.

I became an adept spy, pushing back the curvaceous coffee plant leaves, which look like voluptuous ficus tree leaves. In the closely planted rows, branches brushed against me from all sides, from my toes to my neck, each requiring careful examination. To pick the lower branches, I had to crouch or get down on my knees. All the labor is hands and fingers—no shears or knives, as are used for grapes.

Even more maddening, the cherries along one branch or within the same cluster don't ripen at the same time, and McAlpin insists that pickers pass over the unripe cherries, which in most cases are yellow and olive green. Yellow cherries dappled with red, called *pinton* ("painted"), are acceptable. Dark brown or black cherries that have dried on the tree are also picked, to be separated out at the processing mill. It would be much easier just to strip the branches, but wasting so many cherries that could be picked ripe is unthinkable: McAlpin is selling choice beans, and he sends workers back for three and often four pickings over the course of a few days or weeks. If I wasn't careful to leave the green and yellow cherries, I would have to pick them out of my basket before I was paid; McAlpin pays guest workers just like everybody else.

I popped cherries of varying degrees of ripeness into my mouth to see how they tasted. The translucent goop, called *miel* ("honey"), of both red cherries and *pintons* is sweet and somewhat refreshing, with the taste of overripe melon or fresh litchi nuts. At La Minita, I tasted the hardened *miel* of cherries that had dried on the tree by accident; it tasted like carob. The best flavor came from deep vermilion cherries verging on a mahogany color—the color of dead-ripe Bing cherries. McAlpin told me that this color indicates the height of ripeness, and if it were possible, he would pick only these. But after a day or two, cherries so ripe will begin to dry out and lose flavor, and it is risky to assume that enough workers will be free to pick all of them at the right time.

The beans themselves, which pop out of the cherry with a simple squeeze, are another story. They are a celadon green, rubbery and slimy. The idea of chewing on them the way you would a lozenge or hard candy seems unappealing. But Africans do just that, boiling beans from unripe cherries with herbs and then drying them. Certainly the caffeine would provide more energy than the sugar did from the *miel* I chewed on.

Hopelessly slow, I dreamed of mechanical pickers, which are used on huge farms, typically at low altitudes where robusta grows and price is all. The flatter terrain of these farms allows vibrating machines to pass between rows of trees, shaking the branches until most of the berries fall to the ground. I dreamed even of picking in Kenya, where the trees are higher but are often severely pruned on the side that gets less sun: at least the cherries would be arrayed before me, and I wouldn't have to be a bean scout.

Payday

After an hour, I had a little over a quarter of a basket, which amounted to about a gallon. For my labor, I was solemnly paid thirty cents. Discouraged, I visited several of the pay stations that are set up right along the road, where workers gather at about three P.M., having begun work at sunup. At the height of the harvest, there can be as many as 650 workers, who come from all over the country and live in temporary housing on the plantation. Many Indian families return year after year.

At the station I visited, I saw dozens of teenage boys and girls and a handful of people old enough to be their parents. Many of the boys and men stuffed bandannas into the backs of baseball caps to protect their necks from the sun. Some wore aprons fashioned from cut-up coffee sacks. The footwear was black rubber waders or sneakers or work boots. Dogs who had spent the morning foraging in the ground cover waited for their masters to be paid.

While picking, a worker carries his or her own lightweight sack, into which he or she empties each strapped-on basket as the hours wear on. At the pay station, the workers empty their sacks onto burlap mats. Others join in to pick out the green cherries, twigs and leaves; the green cherries will be bagged separately and used for Costa Rican consumption.

Everyone watches carefully as the cleaned cherries are poured into *cajuelas,* 20-liter (about 5-gallon) square metal containers, each about the size of a milk crate, painted rust red. A year-round La Minita worker smooths the top of each container before emptying it into a communal sack, silently keeping track of each picker's number of containers. "Four and a half," he will call out to another worker holding a cash box, or "six and one," meaning six and one-quarter *cajuelas.*

The man at the pay station seemed as stingy in rounding up to the next quarter-container as the man counting my basket had been. It's his job to conserve the plantation's money, of course, but each full container represents a lot of work. At the time of my visit, the rate happened to correspond to about $1.50 per container, although the price is not tied to the dollar. A typical day's wage was $10 to $20, considered a decent day's pay in a country whose cost of living is far lower than America's. McAlpin says that he pays among the highest wages for farm labor in the country, because the work is so hard, and that Costa Rica's standard of living is envied by its neighbors, as is its democratic system of government, the oldest in Central America.

I watched enviously as one picker after another presented cleaned sacks that filled six, seven or nine containers. Once in a great while, the top picker at La Minita fills fifty baskets in a day, equal to about forty milk-crate *cajuelas*. Clearly, he is material for the annual national picking tournament, with contests for men and for women and rounds of semifinals and finals on various farms. The grand prize is a three- or four-bedroom house of about a thousand square feet. Whoever wins it really earns it.

Like any sizable plantation, La Minita is a world unto itself, with half the year-round work force of eighty and their families living in new, pleasant housing. McAlpin prides himself on the benefits he provides: high wages, matching contributions to a savings plan, private medical care for serious illnesses, a dental clinic, grocery staples at wholesale plus transport, free vegetables from the farm's large garden.

In other countries, however, coffee pickers are frequently not paid fair wages or given anything akin to this range of benefits. Several American-based organizations, such as Coffee Kids and Equal Exchange, seek to ensure that workers are better paid and treated more equitably. Many coffee bars in America ask customers to give their change to one of these groups, collecting it, appropriately enough, in a coffee can.

Even McAlpin, who is faring better than the owners of farms near La Minita, sells coffee from other farms in Costa Rica, Colombia, Guatemala and Sumatra to help support his progressive practices. Most landowners have also had to find some other way to generate income. The 1989 collapse of the International Coffee Agreement, a pact that obliged farmers to hold back supplies in order to keep prices comparatively high, has hurt large and small coffee-producing countries alike. Prices fell to near record lows, because countries no longer sold beans according to prearranged quotas. Efforts to form a new cartel failed. These attempts must continue, though, to ensure the survival of many coffee-producing farms around the world.

Already farms around La Minita are letting jungle overtake some of their coffee trees—a process that can take as little as two years. Farmers who can't afford the labor costs are offering their land to McAlpin at bargain prices. McAlpin himself is subject to many of their difficulties, though, and can by no means afford to take them up on their offers.

Tallying the Harvest

Once paid, the picker puts his or her bills and change into a pocket, collects dog, basket and sack, straps on the backpack that carried the day's food and water, and walks home. When the last picker has been paid, the workers running the pay station fold up the stray sacks, take away the *cajuela*, and group the communal sacks at the roadside to await pickup by one of the farm's tractors. The tractors slowly work their way up the twenty-five miles of roads on the farm, grunting around every bend in the furrowed dirt road so they don't spill any of the beans that are heaped in the trailers. Their destination is the *recibidor*, a blue tin-roofed shed where, throughout the late afternoon and evening, the day's harvested cherries are unloaded, measured and held until dark, when Mack trucks then take them to the processing mill.

The small shed is crowded. When I visited, the two men overseeing the activity were Miguel Morales, the farm manager, and a man who worked at the processing mill. The tractors back up to the front of the shed, which is set into a slope with a road at the front and back. Several men help lift the trailers, whose hydraulic systems are far from springy, in order to disgorge the contents. The driver grabs a shovel and leaps into the tilted trailer to help push out the cherries.

The mill employee, using his hands, guides the fruit into a 200-liter container about the size of a footlocker. Working with practiced motions, he makes a cavity in the center with his hands and pushes the cherries up the sides, the way a baker fills a loaf pan with batter. The exact amount matters: the driver will be held accountable if it doesn't tally with the volume of cherries recorded at the pay station. To measure the final, incomplete portion, he plunges a metal ruler into the heaped cherries and records the level, both on paper and by moving a peg along a wooden board.

When the rust-red container is filled with a load of bright red and yellow cherries, the worker pulls a lever that opens the bottom, and a man waiting in the holding area below shovels the cherries toward the back wall to make room for the next load. By evening, the man will be working atop ten feet of cherries. Visitors can't resist leaping into the huge mound of ripe red cherries, as happy as Charlie in the chocolate factory. The moment is not complete until someone snaps a picture.

At the height of the harvest, the last tractor doesn't unload its cargo until very late, and then all the measured cherries must be reloaded into trucks bound for the processing mill. By the time the tired men push the rest of the day's cherries into the trucks, slogging through the pool of *miel* left on the floor of the shed, it can be near midnight. Still, each night Morales writes down the total figure of the cherries picked on the farm and stops by the hacienda to present it to McAlpin and chat about the day's work over a Coca-Cola. As they talk, the men can usually hear the rumble of the last Mack truck traveling very, very slowly to the mill.

Washing the Beans

The driver of the truck is likely to encounter a number of other similarly filled trucks on the zigzag way to the *beneficio,* as each mill is called. The mills work late into the night because the cherries can't wait: the sweet pulp will start to ferment, and the farmer needs to control that ferment, just as a vintner must harness the fermentation in ripe harvested grapes. In contrast to wine, however, the fermentation of coffee cherries is meant only to loosen the pulp of the fruit from the seeds it holds—the coffee beans—and not to add any flavor. If the beans taste of ferment (and often they do), their value is reduced to virtually zero.

Costa Rican coffees are now considered among the world's best, not just because of the altitude and the soil they grow in but also because of the unusually careful and expensive "wet" processing they undergo. This elaborate treatment is reserved for fine coffees, which means arabicas. A few farmers in search of higher esteem and prices are paying to have their robustas washed, but virtually all robustas (and many lesser-quality arabicas too) are "dry-" or "natural-" processed in areas where water is contaminated, scarce, expensive or all three.

McAlpin derides anyone who likes natural-processed coffees as someone who grew up enjoying mud pies. But his opinion is by no means universal. Many discerning tasters look for and enjoy the taste of dry-processed beans, which they say have an earthy power that washed coffees, however pure and glorious, can never have. (See Chapter Seven, "Coffee by Country," for descriptions of the great coffees of Yemen, the original Mochas; they are always unwashed, as are the sought-after Ethiopian Harrars.)

Mills for the wet process must not be too far from coffee farms, because timing is crucial. Before many hours pass, the skin of the fruit must be removed. "Depulping," as the skinning stage is misleadingly called (the pulp stays, the skin goes), is a Rube Goldberg setup involving sluices of cherries racing up, down and sideways. The seeming confusion, however, is far from casual—the bean's path is carefully planned. Water and gravity guide the whole process, and because the cherries and beans remain in prolonged contact with water, the quality of the water itself is very important. McAlpin recently bought his own mill, on the edge of his farm, which uses water from the Tarrazu River.

As each truck arrives, it unloads the cherries into the same kind of red measuring container as at the farm shed for a final tally of shipments recorded by farm and mill. The fruit immediately plunges into a tank of water. Every cherry that is overripe, brown and shriveled floats to the top and goes into a separate channel, never to be seen again.

The beans that aren't good enough for export, like the underripe beans that don't even make it out of the farm, stay home. It is striking that in many coffee-producing countries, you are just as likely to receive a cup of instant coffee as a brew obsessively measured and steeped in a plunger pot. A typical cup of coffee in Costa Rica is pretty bad, as it is in every coffee-producing country: the crop is grown for export, and the good stuff goes where it fetches the highest price. (The exception is Hawaii, where the crop is so small that growers can fetch high prices from tourists who drink it where it is grown.) McAlpin defends this seemingly unfair system by pointing out that by law, around 11 percent of the country's coffee production must stay within Costa Rica at a regulated low price—the case in many but by no means all coffee-producing countries.

The heavy, good fruit is siphoned to the depulper, a machine not much wider than a person and half as tall. Workers keep their distance from the depulpers: nobody wants to get a finger caught in one. The cherries cascade into a V-shaped opening in which one side is a slanted breastplate and the other a rotating copper-sheathed rasp that tears off the skin. Anyone who has hand-cranked a peeler for Italian plum tomatoes would recognize this machine. As with a tomato peeler, the skin is dumped out the back; it is shoveled off to be turned into mulch. The stripped beans go out the front into a water channel.

The whole mess—seeds encased in their translucent sticky pulp, smaller cherries that escaped with their skin intact, a few whole cherries—courses down to the next odd machine, the first of a series of *cribas* ("sieves"), long rotating cylindrical grates that look like hamster cages. The purpose of the *criba* is to sort by size and keep back the empty skins. The biggest beans go out the first *criba;* smaller whole cherries are pushed along to two more sets of depulpers and *cribas.* Bigger beans command higher prices. They usually signify the ripest and best fruit, although not always.

The endpoint for the skinned cherries is a *pila,* or "trough," a big stone open-topped fermenting tank where the fruit at last comes to rest. Overhead pipes dump the wet beans into separate tubs, by size. The water drains out the bottom, and the seeds sit for anywhere from eight to forty-eight hours or even longer while the sugary mucilage begins to ferment and decompose. A walk past a row of full *pilas* is like a stroll through a farm in the late fall when the smell of silage is strong—at once sour and sweet, like sauerkraut. In dry-processing, fermentation takes place outdoors, either on raised racks or on the ground, where dirt and manure may intrude; then the dry husk is broken and the mucilage scraped off.

Fermentation is necessary at this early stage of processing—but the smell should never be apparent in brewed coffee, even though it frequently is. In a short time, it changes to a sourish off odor. The changeover insidiously becomes apparent hours past the point of no return—when the fermentation has already penetrated the beans themselves, which will have the taste of rotten fruit and even a sweaty onion flavor. It is vital, then, to stop the fermentation at just the right point—when the mucilage comes off easily between the fingers. But there's no setting a timer, because beans will ferment faster or slower in warmer or cooler weather.

This is why the decision to start washing the fermented mucilage off the beans is left to an experienced worker. A good mill will keep staff on duty twenty-four hours, so that when it's time, the washing can start. Others merely stop fermentation at a safe point so the washing coincides with sunlit working hours. The flaw is that the safe point they choose is often too soon: the mucilage won't come off completely, and the beans will have an unpleasantly fruity taste.

The removal of the fermented mucilage takes place in a long, elevated, shallow channel, about a foot wide and 20 inches deep, extending as far as hundreds of feet. In the washing channel, the beans are further separated by size. Doing this requires visual acuity. A worker stands astride the channel wielding a paddle that looks something like a long pizza peel, expertly shunting the beans into various holding tanks by opening or closing gates. Fixed overhead paddles, like the agitator in a washing machine, keep the beans constantly stirred up. The lightest beans flow out soonest, as do those that remained unskinned, unripe or damaged. At the end, the densest *primera* ("first-quality") beans make their way down the channel. The washed and sorted beans flow into stone draining pools, where they remain until they lose their excess water.

Even Drying and an Eagle Eye

Beans in their parchment—a hard, thin jacket that remains once the mucilage is washed away—look something like small pistachio nuts, with a clear tan color that shines in the sun. As the quality decreases, the color of the parchment darkens. One of the holding tanks is usually reserved for brown and black beans, called *borras,* which are used for national consumption. Now the beans must dry, either in the sun or in a mechanical dryer or in a combination of both. If they remain wet, secondary fermentation, which will impart undesirable flavors, can begin.

Sun-drying may sound like the better, more natural way, but mechanical drying offers better control. Sun-drying is certainly the more romantic way. The beans are spread out on patios in big rectangles to a depth of about four or five inches. For seven days to two or three weeks, a worker constantly rakes the beans into checkerboard patterns, going up and down and then across and back. Each big square is like a mini desert, the constantly shifting pattern like shifting sands. Appealing and visually hypnotic as this method is, it won't work in the rain or in cloudy weather or if there isn't enough patio room. And there's no telling what kind of dirt can creep in, or whether morning dew will interrupt the drying, or whether beans at the edges will overdry. The constant tread of the man with the rake doesn't do the beans much good either. Some buyers insist on sun-dried coffee, believing it to have a more interesting flavor, and in the many parts of the world where there is no alternative, research continues into ways of improving the process—drying on concrete versus clay patios, for instance.

More often, though, a mill foreman who has the choice will decide according to weather and available space to send some of the parchment-covered beans to a big rotating drum dryer, where they spin for two or three days at a temperature of between 122 and 140 degrees F. The low temperature is essential for even drying, and so is an eagle eye, because readiness is judged by color. If the beans are not dried long enough and remain too moist, they will absorb air and stale quickly. If they are dried too hot or too long, they will shatter at a touch, spoiling much of their market value. It can take as long as seventy-two hours for the humidity level to descend from 65 or 70 percent moisture to 11 or 12 percent. The very last minutes are crucial, because in just twenty minutes, the beans can lose one percent humidity—and that can be one percent too much.

To tell if the beans are ready, the worker takes a healthy handful of twenty or so and crushes them between his palms. This is like crushing nuts with your hands, and for the beginner, the results are about as dismal. The parchment is stubborn, and comes off, when it does, in jagged shards. A rule of sore thumb is that if six beans in twenty look a little underdone—if the color of the bean is a deep blue verging on black rather than the green verging on straw that is desirable—the whole batch is ready to be poured out of the dryer.

The dried beans, looking more than ever like pistachios, rest in their protective parchment, either in silos or laid on plywood and covered with canvas, until they are shipped. During this *reposo,* which should last a minimum of twenty or thirty days, the humidity is evenly redistributed throughout the bean. The cell structure hardens, and the beans become more resistant to potential damage from humidity or pressure. The rest period for McAlpin's coffee is never longer than six months, because he insists on shipping it before the rains start in earnest, in June.

Polishing the Beans

When an order comes, the parchment is "peeled" off the bean in a machine that works by friction. The first time I saw a sample of highly polished iridescent blue-green beans, I assumed that they must be of high quality. They stood out from the other green beans beside them, which were typically dull and speckled with white. McAlpin, however, prefers matte beans that display a fair amount of silverskin, the lightly glistening, papery chaff that remains beneath the parchment. Even if beans with some silverskin are less comely, he says, the less friction that is applied to them, the less they will break down and release volatile flavor components.

I had naively thought, too, that a gleam was a sign of perfection. Instead, it is a classic mark of underripe beans—a defect that McAlpin calls the most common and overlooked in coffee processing by far. You can recognize underripe beans by looking at the silverskin. On a ripe bean, it will adhere in flaky-looking pieces, whereas on an unripe bean, it will be finely webbed, as if the bean had been sandblasted.

The stripped beans pass over vibrating screens that separate them by size, which is how brokers sell them. McAlpin favors a screening machine from Scotland, manufactured early in the century. Tall, narrow, barn red, with little wood-and-glass doors, it looks like a charming relic. He says that it is more accurate than anything being produced today, and gentler on beans than today's faster machines.

In high-tech mills, the beans then whoosh down long plastic tubes in which they are sorted in machines that use beams of light to check for discolored beans, which could indicate ferment and other defects, against preprogrammed color charts. When a bad bean is detected, a little spurt of air at the base of the tube shoots the bean into a reject tube. Some roasters, like Illy Caffè, in Italy, give each shipment of green beans another sorting.

A Final Sort

La Minita coffee, the only one of the half-dozen coffees McAlpin sells that he names for the whole plantation, goes through an extraordinary final step. Perched on stools in front of partitioned wooden workstations, sixty or seventy women hand-sort the beans, separating out those with adherent silverskin that indicates they are not ripe, and discarding those that are misshapen or discolored. The women work for no more than six hours at a time, with frequent breaks, because the required concentration is so great. The approved beans are double-sewn into big bags.

The sight of a small, brightly lit room full of women poring over green coffee beans one by one seems out of another century. McAlpin admits that light and screen sorters can achieve much of this separation, especially if the beans are fed through slowly and the process is repeated. So far, though, a single machine cannot sort out underripe, discolored and overripe beans at the same time, or make a judgment call on a bean that is only partially flawed. McAlpin says that he's in the business of creating jobs, and this one is relatively pleasant: clean and with minimal supervision from a man who goes up and down the aisles to see that the "good" beans really are good. I was assured that when visitors aren't present to look over the women's shoulders, the conversation is nonstop and the music from the radio loud.

The journey from the final sorting room to the hometown specialty-coffee shop is surprisingly short. A bag of coffee from Costa Rica can reach a broker or roaster in a port city in under three weeks and, with land transport, can get from Costa Rica to almost any city or town in little over a month. Shipping takes longer from countries that are farther from the United States, but the general method is the same: in bags loaded into containers. The thick metal housing of the container usually ensures that odors from other cargo will not contaminate the beans, but not always. McAlpin has had disasters, like the time the smell of untreated rubber in a neighboring container invaded the beans he was shipping—luckily, not La Minita beans. "It was like the inside of new shoes," McAlpin says. "Gross."

Today, synthetic substitutes for burlap are used for the bags; before they came into use, an off-smelling coating could affect the coffee, leading to an old, "baggy" taste.

Compared to the all-important role that soil, climate, careful tending and processing play, though, transport is responsible for few taste defects. This is a lucky thing. A coffee farmer puts his skill into and risks his livelihood on each year's crop, and he wants his beans to be at their best when they reach their destination. When they do, they will undergo the inspection that will determine not only their fate but the farmer's as well.

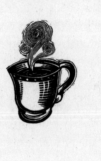

CHAPTER TWO 2 | Cupping

THE MOMENT OF TRUTH FOR A BEAN and all the people who helped grow, process and ship it comes with cupping—a ritualized evaluation of coffee beans performed behind the scenes, first by bean brokers (importers) and then by the companies, large and small, the broker sells to. An entire country's coffee tastes are formed in the cupping room, whether by experts at a huge conglomerate who decide what to buy for supermarket blends or by your neighborhood coffee fanatic turned coffee roaster.

Cupping follows a peculiar, precise procedure codified more than a hundred years ago. The brewing method—steeping—resembles that used for tea. The brew it produces would not bring a smile to the lips of a coffee lover. A very few beans are roasted so light that most people would be repelled by the sour brew they produce; a carefully weighed amount of the roasted beans is steeped in an equally carefully measured volume of hot water in handleless cups or low glasses. Tasters wait for the grounds to settle and the liquid to cool to a temperature most drinkers would find uninvitingly tepid, and then they sniff, slurp and spit with a complete lack of decorum. Professional cuppers have tasted thousands of beans during their careers, and they usually go through bean samples so fast that the classic furniture for a cupping room is a rotating table. The taster jerks it around with shocking velocity, methodically slurping and spitting like some machine gone awry, all the while hurriedly scrawling scores on a strange-looking score sheet.

This Charlie Chaplinesque scene takes place most often in the cupping room at a brokerage house, where hundreds of beans must be dispatched in a single morning, or at a big commercial company. Brokers and big companies are looking to reject only coffee so terrible they just can't use it. Their tolerance for second- and third-rate beans is broad. Brokers usually want to sell as much as they can, and with a quick taste they can decide the most suitable potential market or whether the sample is completely hopeless. Big companies need to buy a lot of beans at a time, and their goal is consistency rather than excellence; they want to find beans that will keep up their signature blends as cheaply as possible.

The pace in the cupping room of an average specialty roaster doesn't match the speeded-up-movie pace typical of a big company or broker. ("Roaster" here means not a piece of equipment but a person who chooses and roasts beans.) It is rarely leisurely, however. Even a medium-sized coffee roaster isn't usually on the lookout for magnificence: the idea is to find something usable, generally for a blend, and this can require plowing through a good many samples sent by brokers. No one would mind being surprised by greatness, of course, while tasting through the day's batch. But no one expects it.

The thin and astringent brew is designed not to be enjoyed but to be used to diagnose defects and, secondarily, quality. The light roast also reveals the bean's acidity in its widest possible range. Acidity is not a defect. Most of the flavor and delicacy of a bean is in its acids, even if the word "acid" sounds harsh. This distinctiveness will bring a higher price, and so it must be accentuated by both the seller and the buyer; a dark roast blunts acidity, and a really dark roast can obliterate it. (For a full discussion of coffee acids and the crucial role they play in flavor, see Chapter Three, "Roasting.") Besides revealing acidity, a light roast challenges a bean to show how much body it really has; a darker roast will coat the tongue better than a light one, making the beans seem more substantial. And even though the aroma is breathed in through every facial pore as soon as the hot water goes over the grounds, the wait for a cool cup enables a far more accurate diagnosis than would drinking the liquid hot. The steeped brew on a cupping table, then, however strange it might seem to an ordinary coffee drinker, allows a taster to separate out and consider each of the categories by which beans are judged: acid, body and overall aroma and flavor.

Why not just roast a sample of green beans to a standard degree and taste it like a normal person? If a roaster wants to sell a bean "straight," or unblended, this is, indeed, a logical next step after a cupping. The roaster will sip away and pretend to be a customer. But usually a taster is looking for something specific—body to beef up a blend, say, or acid to sharpen the blend's flavor. Cupping is the best means to determine which beans will have the desired effect.

A Taste of Things to Come

The atmosphere was tense the morning I visited The Coffee Connection to eavesdrop on a cupping of Guatemalan, Costa Rican and Kenyan coffees. The small, sterile room at the company's headquarters, in an industrial section of Boston, was windowless and sheathed top to bottom in white Formica. It looked like a laboratory—typical for a cupping room, which is supposed to be a sensory-isolation chamber.

The passion of The Coffee Connection's founder, George Howell, awakened much of the Northeast to what fine coffee could taste like; with Peet's, its West Coast counterpart, it long stood as the country's leading example of a high-quality medium- to large-scale roaster. (In 1994, Howell sold the chain of several dozen stores to Starbucks. He recently opened Copacafé, his own coffeehouse in Lexington, Massachusetts, and began GHH Select, a mail-order company selling beans that live up to his standards and philosophy.) Howell became legendary for doing anything to find clean, beautifully processed beans: for years he maintained first call on the best La Minita beans, grown by his close friend Bill McAlpin.

And this early morning, McAlpin himself is present in the cupping room, having driven six hours the night before from his home in Bar Harbor, Maine.

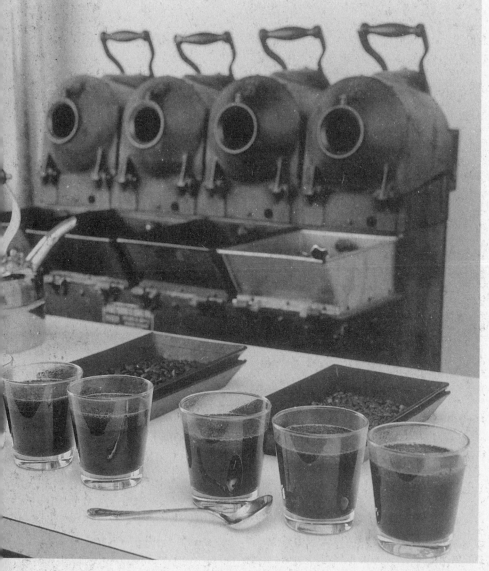

Sample roaster and cupping table

La Minita beans, a known quantity, are not under scrutiny. Instead, the two men are meeting to judge samples procured by McAlpin in his secondary role as broker. McAlpin has also brought along another Costa Rican coffee of his own for Howell to taste for use in a blend. But the chief business of the morning is Guatemala.

Howell has been perplexed by the poor quality of the season's beans from the city of Antigua—considered by many to be the site of the best Guatemalan coffees. Along with La Minita and certain Kenyan coffees, Antiguan and other Guatemalan beans elicit awe from coffee men like Howell, but not the ones he'd had lately. Every single shipment is different, even if the name is the same, because it might have come from a different processing mill or have had a bad trip from the producing country or, heaven forbid, it might even be "past crop"—last year's harvest, kept sitting around a warehouse while it lost its vigor and fresh flavor. A vigilant roaster tastes any lot before committing to buy it from a broker or roast it for customers.

It is very rare for a broker to be present when a roaster, his customer, samples beans: seller and buyer usually maintain relations that are both cordial and wary. Everything is done by overnight mail, fax and phone. The roaster scores the brewed sample beans by several criteria, some universal and some idiosyncratic, and then faxes the broker: "Ship me as many bags as you've got" (bag sizes vary, but average 150 pounds) or, in effect, "One zippered sandwich bag was more than enough, thank you."

Painstaking quality control is especially important before an order is placed. Often, the sacks of coffee beans arrive, and when the roaster cups a sample of the beans first thing on a roast day, they don't taste anything like they did months ago at the cupping. Careful roasters keep back some of the green beans from the original cupping-day sample, for purposes of comparison. Savvy ones sign order contracts on an "SAS" basis, meaning "same as shipped." Otherwise, it is difficult to make a broker take back faulty shipments, and invariably the effort will mean lost freight charges. Better to be careful sooner and avoid disputes later.

A roaster can eliminate some samples by sight. Pinprick holes can be a mark of insect infestation, leaving the bean hollow and lightweight and creating a woody taste. Black spots where fruit flies left deposits of acid will impart a dirty flavor; so will mold resulting from drying that took place too slowly. "Elephant ears" are two coffee cherries that have grown around each other rather than apart, forming a big, hollow bean. Just because beans look shriveled or brownish doesn't mean there's anything wrong with them, though. Unwashed, or "natural-processed," beans usually look this way. But a frankly black bean can be a dreaded fungus-infected "stinker," and it can ruin a whole batch.

Once a cupping sample has been looked over, roasting it is no simple task. Because the quantity is so small, the beans are heated in a special "sample roaster," which looks like two or three adjacent mini missiles over a gas flame (gas roasters are the most common; there are also electric ones). Each missile has an inner cylinder that spins over the flame, and each can be tilted to dump the beans onto a narrow perforated tray to cool quickly. Mastering the miniature world of sample roasters requires its own set of reflexes. This falls to the person who usually operates a regular-sized commercial roaster and is familiar with their pitfalls, many of which can also occur in a sample roaster. (These machines are too expensive and impractical for most home kitchens, and they require extensive ventilation.)

Once the beans are roasted and cooled, they are ground medium-coarse and spooned into the bottom of each cup. The industry rule is an exact 7.25 grams of coffee (the weight of a nickel and a dime) to 5 ounces (⅔ cup) of water. To simplify what could be a very tedious process, many companies that regularly hold cupping sessions duplicate the standard measurements recommended for brewing: 1 coffee scoop, which equals 2 tablespoons, to 6 ounces (¾ cup) of water.

Part Men's Club, Part Lab

When rigged out, a cupping room resembles something between a high-school chemistry lab and a private club. The lab part is the rows of low glass cups, which look like juice glasses (and often are), lined up dangerously near the edges of the tables. The men's club part is the blue or billiard-table-green leatherette trays for the beans. Generally there are at least two trays per kind of bean, one to show the green beans and one to show them roasted. A third tray might show the grind; Robert Dattala, formerly master roaster for The Coffee Connection, lays out grind samples in neat long rectangles about the shape of cigarettes. Tasters are supposed to be able to see everything at a glance—except the handwritten label identifying the sample. Tastings are "blind," so that preconceptions will not cloud judgment.

Also part of the club look is the sterling-silver tasting spoons that experienced tasters wield, the way sommeliers dangle hammered-silver tasting cups as they tell people which wine to order. The spoons, sometimes engraved with the taster's name and featuring elaborate chased designs, are not just badges of status. Silver absorbs and dissipates heat (think of your mother telling you to put a sterling spoon into a glass before pouring in a hot liquid); silver plate will serve the same purpose. The bowls of the spoons are wide and shallow, like soup spoons, to allow the liquid to cool fast and mix with oxygen. Mixing oxygen into anything you're tasting brings out the flavors. This is the point of the indecorous noises tasters of any liquid make when they slurp and slosh.

A taster samples several cups made from the same beans. The minimum is three, and if the beans are particularly important—meaning expensive, or the basis of a signature blend—the taster will insist on six cups. Just a few specks of coffee grounds from a bad bean in a sample batch can make the difference between a "clean cup" and a "dirty cup," meaning one that is defect-free and one that shows defects. The more cups per sample, the greater the chance that the roaster will recognize any problems with the beans on offer.

As with all tasting rituals, it's good to have eaten a wide variety of foods for taste references. It's also good to have sniffed deeply or, better, to have put into your mouth a number of things you shouldn't have: rotten apples and spoiled chicken soup and yogurt, raw potatoes and their peels, underripe bananas, tomato soup, overcooked hard-boiled eggs (preferably kept too long in the refrigerator), cardboard, paper bags, Styrofoam and, even more useful, wood, straw, hay and dirt.

Tasters may all have similar standards, but they rarely use the same words to describe them. The problem is that there isn't an adjective for "brown paper bag" or "raw potato," and every expert comes up with his or her own flavor descriptions. Wine writers may spout words they have no business using, but at least they have created a vocabulary. Leaders of the coffee world, for example, Ted Lingle, of the Specialty Coffee Association of America, have tried to build from scratch a lexicon to describe flavor attributes. The confusing and contradictory terms—one man's "grassy" is another man's "floral," one man's "blueberry" another's "old tomato soup"—are a notorious example of why the coffee world often resembles the Tower of Babel.

"The Nose Does the Work"

Howell arrives late to the early-morning cupping, having been caught in terrible traffic. He's under pressure. A group of Coffee Connection store managers and interested Bostonians are waiting in the next room for him to give a lecture and slide presentation on the raising of coffee, and the intercom doesn't stop squawking with various urgent pages. McAlpin, generally a placid man, becomes agitated: a lot is riding on Howell's ability to concentrate on these coffees. After Howell responds to the third page, McAlpin says, "Relax, George. I drove six hours for this."

Dattala begins to pour hot, but not boiling, water into the cups. The ideal water temperature is around 210 degrees F—just below the boil, so that unnecessarily bitter substances won't be extracted. For a while, nobody moves. The grounds are exciting themselves, milling around the hot water, fizzing slightly as they release carbon dioxide formed while roasting. Within a minute or two, they have floated to the top and formed a thickish dome over the cup. Iridescent blue bubbles appear like oil on macadam.

The first task is "breaking the crust"—plunging a spoon into the grounds domed at the top to get a strong reading of the beans. The taster bends to put his or her nose right over the cup. Fragrant steam bathes the face, and sometimes coffee grounds do too. The aromas that rush out give a powerful and frequently seductive impression of the coffee. Alfred Peet, who helped revive American interest in good coffee, says that "the nose does the work," and when you break the crust, you see what he means. The light, singing notes of acid appear, and so do sweeter, darker notes. So strong is the bouquet that you can believe you've learned everything right away. The first impression, though, can be a siren song.

Some defects do make themselves plain at the outset. The commonest is ferment, which smells like something you kept in the refrigerator way too long. Ferment in beans is the result of enzymatic activity during improper storage (different from the essential ferment that during initial processing eases the removal of the seeds from the pulp of the fruit), and nothing good comes of it. Ferment can't be hidden by roasting or otherwise masked, unlike other defects that don't necessarily come across to the coffee drinker as something wrong. Buyers are especially alert to it, because ferment will get stronger as the roast gets darker. While Howell is on the phone, McAlpin smells a fermented sample on the table, from a sample he didn't bring. He asks Dattala to take all six cups away. "I don't want George's tastes to get screwed up," he says.

Howell, McAlpin and Dattala each break the crusts of one of the three cups Dattala has laid out for each sample, silently noting their first reactions. They're far too respectful to blurt out what they think, and each knows that he will learn more about his own opinion by waiting to discuss it with the others. Dattala then goes down the line carrying a big old-fashioned kettle, topping up each cup to encourage the grounds to sink. Then whoever feels like it chips in to skim off the light tan scum that floats to the top of each cup, wielding two shallow soup spoons like the paddles of a canoe and jettisoning the scum into an empty glass.

The Moment of Truth

The part that counts—the tasting—is a noisy, impolite business. The goal is to cover all at once the parts of the tongue that register the four basic tastes —sour, sweet, bitter, salty—at the same time mixing in as much oxygen as possible. This is done by inhaling the coffee in one vacuuming sip that pulls the liquid all the way to the back of the tongue. (The grounds that have not been skimmed remain safely at the bottom of the cup.) The idea is to mount a surprise attack on the palate, jolting the olfactory senses into giving a perfectly true account. Then comes loud sloshing and spitting.

Pleasure is not an official part of the plan, although unexpected flavors can be powerfully pleasurable. These usually come only to those who wait. A nice warming draught is almost the worst way to taste, first because it's easy to burn your tongue. The important undertones appear as the coffee cools.

At the beginning, sweetness and body will be clear, but acids will be muted. If they don't come into focus as the liquid cools, the coffee is usually old. Aged beans can be richly mellow but also just plain dull, robbed of their winy snap by too much time in a warehouse. As the coffee cools, a kind of dead woodiness can enter, another sign of faulty processing. In Kenyan and other East African coffees, this can be read as a black-pepper taste, and

George Howell once thought the pepper flavor desirable in those coffees. Now he calls it a defect—a sign of age he finds in other coffees, too, even if roasters pass off the beans, as he once did, as "spicy."

Another common defect is called "Rio-y," because it was so frequently found in Brazilian beans shipped through Rio de Janeiro. It is also called "hard." No one is sure what causes the flavor, which tastes like iodine. Is it fertilizers? Chemical-laden sea breezes? Bacteria? Molds? Fungi? Ted Lingle says that it results from too many sour, undesirable acids and not enough sugars or salts, and comes across as a "stinging, sour sensation." Although most professionals avoid Rio-y coffee, some countries—notably Turkey—actually prefer it, having grown accustomed to it over many decades.

Then there are taints that correspond directly to the troublemaker. If coffee trees have been planted too near rubber trees, as they are in several coffee-producing countries including the Philippines, the coffee tastes just like rubber. This problem can turn up in commercial canned coffee. Beans that dry on the tree before being picked can sometimes also give a rubbery flavor. If beans have been stored in warehouses beside spices like mace, allspice or pepper, there will be incongruous and possibly unpleasant hints in the brew. When coffee bags used to be shipped alongside animal skins destined for the leather trade, the bad taste imparted by the skins acquired its own name: "hidey."

The commonest of the direct defects is earthiness—literally the taste of dirt. Many problems in processing beans can cause this: washing with tainted water, drying that is too slow or too long, storage in a moist or too-warm place. Some roasters find a certain amount of dirt "charming" or "rustic"; any connoisseur of Yemen Mocha Mattari, for instance, practically demands funk, because it is a defining characteristic of that coffee.

Howell wants the finish always to be sweet. He rarely gets his wish, because so many unripe beans find their way into samples. Unripeness reads as an astringent taste, like green bananas. McAlpin's obsession is harvesting and processing coffee to perfection, and he is something of a fanatic about ripe berries. He has helped Howell sort out the difference between lively, desirable acid—which will play against other flavors in a normal roast—and astringent unripeness, which in any roast will be unpleasant. Many tasters attribute the flavor of immaturity to underroasted coffee, which is usually called grassy.

The place to look for underripeness, which McAlpin says is the most commonly undetected coffee defect, is in the finish, about ten seconds after you swallow. Is there the usual combination of mellowness and sharpness and also the sugar of, say, a medium-ripe apple? Or is there in addition a harsh, arid lack of sweetness, as if you'd been robbed of a bit of sugar that the first taste had promised?

Since the focus is so sharply on defects, a cupper's vocabulary practically evaporates when it comes to describing good qualities in coffee. It's easier to describe something you don't like than something you do. Among the few positive terms in the coffee taster's lexicon are "neutral," "mild," "clean," "sweet," "delicate," "fine," "fresh," "full," "rich" and "sound." Roasters develop their own vocabulary for qualities they enjoy and want to find again. Comparisons to chocolate and spices like cinnamon and clove abound, and so do comparisons to popular wines like Burgundy and Chardonnay. George Howell is fixated on what he calls the blackberry flavor of Kenyan coffee.

Surprisingly, flavor suffers little as coffee cools. Tea leaves contain tannin, which begin to impart bitter flavors after five minutes. But brewed coffee is safe, as long as it has been safely removed from a heat source. (The coffee lover's chant should be, "Get that coffee off the burner!") The parade of cups in the cupping room can sit undisturbed for hours as tasters go back and back to slurp another spoonful.

A cupping can be a long or very short procedure. I once helped judge a series of Kenyan coffees at a competition Howell was holding: he would reward the most careful processing factories by paying more for their beans. In each session, it took us as long as two hours to evaluate six coffees, as we kept changing our minds while the coffee cooled. As coffee comes to room temperature, acid and sweet perform a kind of ballet: high notes flatten and recede, and darker, sweeter notes come to the fore.

Most tasters would consider this lengthy contemplation a kind of tortured refinement. The broker who cups hundreds of samples in a day allows plenty of dirty and flawed samples to pass inspection. Experienced brokers are shrewd, though, and know how to appreciate a fine coffee—and what they can charge for it.

The tasting at The Coffee Connection lasts about forty minutes, long in the usual world of sip, spit, jot down a note or two, and order or pass. Howell, at last able to concentrate, admires the Guatemalan Antiguas, which he calls better than the ones he has been shipped lately. McAlpin is visibly relieved: he knows that Howell will place an order, and this means his trip was worth it. His own Costa Rican is of less urgent concern, but he is still very pleased when Howell raves about it. A great Costa Rican coffee has real character, and this is a good one. Howell comes around to the opinion McAlpin expressed several times when Howell was answering pages: "That's the best coffee on the table." Even if everyone has ingested a fair amount of caffeine since the tasting began, the atmosphere in the room is noticeably more relaxed.

Cupping at Home

It's easy enough to arrange a cupping in your own kitchen, even though you probably won't make a habit of it. Brewing coffee in your usual way will give you a better idea if a certain bean is something you'll enjoy drinking. But cupping can be a useful exercise, if only to bury your nose in the vapor when you break the crust.

Start by grinding samples of two or three coffees until they are at a medium grind—like cornmeal or coarse grit. Wipe out the grinder with a damp paper towel before and after grinding each sample. The beans should be roasted to the same degree, which should be as light as you can find. Choose a small array that will best show you differences. You might start out with, say, a Central American like Costa Rica or Guatemala and an Indonesian like Sumatra or Sulawesi. If you can find Kenya or Zimbabwe, you'll be able to judge a high-acid coffee against the other two. Sumatra will have the heaviest body but be light on acid. The Central American should have both acid and body, with stronger acid (remember, the acid in coffee beans means liveliness and sparkle, not stomachaches).

Put 1 coffee scoop, or 2 tablespoons, of each kind of coffee at the bottom of a cup or glass; all the containers should ideally be the same size and have a capacity of 6 to 8 ounces. Advanced cupping would involve two or three cups for each kind of coffee, but that's probably taking things too far. You can look for defects, the way the pros do, and you might well find some; but the real point of the exercise is to learn distinctions between different kinds of coffee. Line up the cups on a counter or table where you'll be able to reach them with ease.

Bring a pot of water to the boil and let it sit for fifteen to thirty seconds, to bring down the temperature to about 210 degrees F. Pour 5 ounces of water into each cup. Measure ½ cup plus 2 tablespoons for the first, and go by eye with the rest, matching the level of the first cup. By the time you've finished pouring, the first cups will have already formed a dome.

You don't have to wait long to break the crust — the fun part. Plunge a soup spoon, preferably silver-plated, into the thick cover of grounds, and bend way over to stick your face into the cup. Bathe your nostrils, your cheeks, your mouth in the steam, and think about what you smell. Is it sour? Sweet? Dry and acrid? Fermented? Brothy? Grassy? Flowery? Spicy? Like clumps of dirt? This smell will be your most powerful experience of the coffee, and if you're being methodical, you can take notes to remember how the first impression compares with the taste of the cooled coffee.

Pour 1 or 2 more tablespoons of water into each cup, so the grounds will all fall to the bottom. Skim off the scum with two spoons, going just beneath the surface to capture the wrinkled light tan foam; toss the foam into an empty cup.

Now wait. The idea is to detect a wider variety of flavors than you find in the usual hot cup of coffee, and the best way is not to try while the coffee is hot: let it cool to at least lukewarm. Then suck up a shallow spoonful of coffee while sucking in air through your nostrils. Don't be afraid to make noise. Think of yourself as a vacuum cleaner. Try to pull the liquid over your tongue, and slosh it around your whole mouth. How's the body — the weight of the liquid on your palate? It should feel as though you have something fuller than water in your mouth. Do the flavors vanish almost before the liquid reaches the back of the throat? Or do they seem to expand and sweeten? Or do you get paper bag instead?

With luck, you won't taste any of the egregious defects a roaster should have weeded out: the pungent, unmistakable, old-sock taste of ferment or Rio-y, chemical-like tastes. But it's likely that you'll have a dirty cup, meaning off flavors unrelated to acid or sweetness, and that you might have the puckering astringency of unripe coffee. (For an example of a whistle-clean coffee, check the Sources, page 251, to order a single-estate Costa Rican coffee. Whether you like it or not, you'll be able to see what a clear, unsullied coffee is. Then you can go back to whatever you prefer.)

Chat, make a phone call or wash some dishes, to let the coffee cool completely. A watched cup seems never to cool, but after fifteen to twenty minutes, the coffee will be at its X-ray clearest. Slurp spoonfuls again and compare notes with your first impressions. At the end, a coffee reveals its strengths and weaknesses, and when it is cool, the acids seem both at their brightest and at their most desirable. You might get lucky and find one so full of flavor that you won't ever want to adulterate it with milk and sugar.

CHAPTER THREE $\Big|$ # Roasting

A COFFEE SHOP'S SUCCESS ultimately rests on the skill and palate of the person who buys and roasts the beans. In contrast to the small army of people who determine the final taste of a wine, in the coffee trade one person—a true "roastmaster"—does everything but nourish and harvest the beans: buys them, decides which ones to combine into a signature blend, and calls on experience and a sixth sense to judge how long and at what temperature to cook them.

A clumsy or distracted roaster (in the coffee business, "roaster" more often means the person who operates the machine than the machine itself) can watch the company's investment go up the smokestack. A skilled and subtle roaster, on the other hand, can transform mediocre beans into a smooth blend and very good beans into something unforgettable.

A green coffee bean is called "raw" for a reason: all the potential flavor is locked inside it. True, a deep whiff of a cupped handful of green beans can predict much about how the roasted bean will taste. But if you brewed raw beans, they would have no recognizable coffee taste. Grinding them would be no easy trick, either: raw beans are compact and tough, whereas after roasting they are brittle and easily crushed.

Fire gives coffee its flavor. The carbohydrates in green beans need to be heated to develop toasty, sweet flavors. Some of the naturally occurring acids are driven off, and other, flavor-making acids are developed. Why roast, rather than use some other cooking method? Other ways either don't develop the flavors at all or don't develop them properly. Boiling water, for instance, isn't hot enough to bring about these changes. Boiling oil is: eighteenth-century travelers to Africa reported seeing people eat deep-fried balls of roasted and ground coffee bound with fat.

No one deep-fries beans today, at least not yet. Aside from the expense and the problems of gumming up coffee grinders and producing greasy cups, the chief impracticalities of cooking beans in fat show why anyone who roasts must be very nervous: during cooking, the temperature must be adjusted depending on the weather and the particular batch (boiling oil is way too hot to be easily controlled); and the process must be stopped, fast, the second the beans are ready. Deep-fried beans would likely be deep-fried charcoal.

Observing the Roast

Roasting at home is a romantic idea. In many Arab countries, stirring beans over an open flame has always begun the coffee ceremony, and in some Latin American households stovetop roasting is still the norm. (The technique is really dry-frying, but all cooking methods commonly used for beans are called "roasting.") For many years in the United States, too, people roasted coffee beans at home. Old devices still turn up at tag sales and flea markets, usually either shallow pans with built-in stirrers, like old-fashioned stovetop popcorn poppers, or metal globes with cranks that spin the beans.

Clearly, many people get the hang of home roasting, but it has always been a disaster for me. First, there is the problem of the initial heat of the pan. I tried several pans, the last one a thin aluminum sauté pan about 1½ inches deep and 8 inches wide that was made in Guatemala. The box, gaily decorated with yellow and red Indian designs, included an oven thermometer to gauge the temperature of the pan and the beans, a flat-bottomed wooden spoon, hand-loomed oven mitts and a tiny burlap sack of green Guatemalan beans. Too bad about the beans. They were the lovely, limpid blue-green of a good high-grown, washed, Central American coffee and deserved better than they got.

The thermometer, whose manufacturer surely would protest this use, registered the recommended 500 degrees F as I began. This temperature, roasters have since informed me, is far too high: at the outset, it should never be more than 425 degrees. As soon as I poured in the beans, they began to scorch on the outside, queering my ability to judge doneness by color—an often misleading guide, but the most common one. The thermometer was useless after the beans went in, thrown off by the temperature of the warm air around the beans and by contact with the beans. From then on, it was seat-of-the-pants roasting, and the final result was such a disastrous combination of green, brown and black beans that I had no desire to brew it.

I do recommend stovetop roasting, though, if only in a junior-high science-experiment way. It will make you familiar with green beans, and it will give you a chance to smell their grassy, earthy, flowery fragrances for yourself. (Many of the companies listed in the Sources, pages 251–52, that mail roasted beans will, on request, mail green beans.) And it lets you watch and smell the changes green beans undergo when they are heated. Just keep the windows open.

Before beans turn brown, they turn a straw yellow or amber. This occurs about two minutes into a roast. Some raw beans, particularly dry-processed "green" beans, are actually a mottled beige or light brown when they are shipped.

A large part of the junior-high fun is to listen to the beans pop. After about five minutes, they begin to swell; the side with the groove running down the middle, called the "center cut," starts out concave and flattens as it expands. Changes in the bean's water content help explain the changes in shape and size. Green beans contain anywhere from 8 to 14 percent water.

The "free water," or plain liquid between the cells, mostly evaporates during the drying of the green beans before they are shipped. The remaining water is chemically bound within the cells and turns to steam as the beans heat; depending on the roast degree, the final water content is about 2 percent. After the interior temperature of the bean exceeds the boiling point, the pressure of water vapor, along with carbon dioxide gas that is produced as carbohydrates decompose, puts stress on the cell walls. Because the walls are pliable, the bean expands rather than bursts.

Even if the bean doesn't explode, it does make a noise just like popping corn, and it nearly doubles in volume. The center cut gets wider and shallower, disgorging papery silverskin, or chaff, which winds like a sail from the outer surface into the bean. Silverskin adhering to the rounded side of the bean, nearly invisible on the green bean, flies off too. If you are watching this closely in a pan on your stove, you will notice chaff waft around the kitchen and settle in remote places—another of the many inconveniences of home roasting. Flecks of chaff also stick to the pan and burn, and are practically impossible to clean. After roasting, you can still see a whitish trail of silverskin along the center cut, and if you break open the bean, you will discover the last furlings. Roasters refer to the loud event by several names: the "first pop"; "12 percent," for the amount of weight lost at that point, mostly through evaporation and the release of carbon dioxide, a heavy gas; and "pyrolysis."

"Pyrolysis" is an important term that properly refers to all the chemical changes that occur when the interior produces heat of its own, not just the first pop. The internal heat breaks down the bean's raw components and forms hundreds of new aromatic volatile compounds—at least eight hundred, according to some sources, such as Bernhard Rothfos, the author of definitive guides to coffee technology. These compounds include aldehydes and ketones, chemicals that flavor wine and most foods, and also tiny concentrations of sulfides, which in higher concentration are obnoxious (rotten eggs, unlit gas) but in very low concentration help define coffee flavor.

The roaster must know exactly what to do as soon as he or she hears the beans start to pop, because so much that will affect the final flavor happens in the next few minutes. The traditional roaster has to make do with the minimal controls on a standard machine. The machine that small or medium-sized specialty roasters typically use is nothing more than a rotating drum with hot air blowing in constantly, like an electric clothes dryer, and interior paddles that continually throw the beans back onto themselves. It looks like an old steam locomotive, and is sometimes enameled a sporty maroon. Green beans are loaded into the top and discharged from a front door at the bottom.

In some early drum roasters, the fire was placed inside the drum, but this was soon abandoned in favor of banks of gas jets running along the length of the bottom of the drum, like the broiler at the bottom of a gas oven. A refinement that conserves heat is to encase the drum in an insulated metal jacket, with a few inches of air between the drum and the jacket. Extremely hot air from below whooshes up between the spinning drum and the stationary jacket and then through the drum. A ventilating fan moves the hot air through an opening in the back and out the drum.

The heat that the gas jets produce must be sufficient to get the mass of beans inside the drum—250 pounds is a typical capacity—well on their way to the first pop. The drum machine employs several kinds of heat: convection, from the hot air passing around the beans; radiant, from the heat emanating from the metal walls of the rotating drum and later from the beans themselves; and direct, from the beans touching the walls and each other. Once the beans are hot, they transfer heat to each other, and the whole process speeds up. A warm drum helps: the day's second roast is always faster and better than the first, the way the second cup of espresso from a good machine always is, and a roastmaster often dismisses an uninteresting bean as "good for heating up the roaster." A warm day helps too. Or a roaster can take the expensive, fuel-consuming step of preheating the machine for as long as forty-five minutes.

Every few seconds after the first pop, the roaster checks a sample of the tumbling beans for their changing size, color, surface texture and smokiness, withdrawing a small scoop from an opening at the front of the drum's housing. If the bean is high-grown, it will be dense, and will require a higher temperature for ideal flavor development. Also, a high-grown bean has more acids than a low-grown bean, and roasters may want to choose a temperature and roast time that will showcase its acidity.

A Welcome Acidity

Acidity is the reason some high-grown arabicas fetch a higher price. All green beans are high in chlorogenic acid (7 percent), which by itself is unpleasantly astringent. As the roast progresses, much of the chlorogenic acid disappears and other, flavorful acids form, more than making up for its loss. These include acids familiar from everyday foods: acetic acid, the kind in vinegar; citric acid, as in citrus fruits; malic acid, which is a pronounced component of apples, grapes and certain wines; and formic acid.

The names might make coffee sound positively corrosive. But the acids we associate with unpleasant sourness form only when brewed coffee is overheated or when beans are underroasted, leaving too much chlorogenic acid. Acids develop nicely as the roast turns medium-dark, but then they break down as a roast gets frankly dark. Espresso roasts are usually brought to a deep brown, so they will be comparatively low in acid. Espresso's brewing method makes the reduction of acid a necessity: at espresso's potent concentration of flavor, a lightish roast highlighting acidity would be intolerable.

Acidity gives a cup much of its complexity, and if there isn't enough of it, coffee loses life and sparkle. Acids make each sip interesting. They make you pay attention to the balance of sensations on the palate—bitter, sweet, tart—and lead you to think about the quality of the beans you bought.

Naturally, there are tradeoffs. A light to medium roast that shows off acids will frequently be light in body, because it lacks many of the caramelized sugars that give body and "mouthfeel" to a darker roast. People become addicted to dark roasts, which connote sophistication and "real coffee" to many. But true sophistication is appreciating the range of roast styles that suit various kinds of beans. The darker the bean, the higher the degree of caramelization. People who like blackened toast crusts, as I do, will savor in a dark roast the flavors caused by browning reactions. These are called "Maillard reactions," and what is browned are the few proteins and many carbohydrates in the beans. When taken too far, though, the carbohydrates produce a burnt taste.

Another tradeoff—and another reason the roaster has to start with a clear idea of how he or she wants the final bean to taste—is that as the beans caramelize and gain body, the heat that just a minute before produced peak flavor starts to reduce acidity. Then the acids are gone forever. If the green beans are high in chlorogenic acid and few other kinds, as robustas are, this loss is no tragedy. But it is a great shame to mute the interesting acids in a superb Central American or East African arabica bean.

A Guide to Roasts

Another decision the roaster must make early is how much oil to let come to the surface. About 15 percent of the substances in green beans are oils, and they are crucial flavor carriers, even if only a tiny fraction of them appear in the final cup (they add negligible calories to the liquid). As cell walls break down during pyrolysis, oil that was chemically bound within the bean is free to move through the newly porous cell walls toward the surface. A few minutes after the first pop, the exhaust gives off a bluish smoke. The bean's oil appears first in tiny droplets, as if through so many pinpricks, and then in noticeable blotches, finally creating a gloss over every part of the surface. By the time a gloss forms, the bean looks blackish.

Roast names are one of the most controversial territories in the coffee world, and they lead to confusion and annoyance. Some roasters despise the very idea of putting names to roasts ("Disinformation," grumbles Jerry Baldwin, the director of Peet's, in the Bay Area), and each roaster seems to have his or her own definition of what a name means. I agree with those who mourn the loss of regional variations in coffee—the preference for one roast style over another in different parts of the country. Calling black-as-tar beans "French" on the West Coast and "Italian" on the East, though, simply out of long-standing usage, helps no one, especially now that so many people mail-order coffee from another part of the country. So here is a rough and general guide to American roast names, with apologies to those who would forever banish them:

Cinnamon Roast: The lightest roast, "cinnamon," is the color of bark cinnamon and has no oil on the surface. Large manufacturers often incorporate very light-roasted coffee into their blends, because roasting for a short time both saves money and adds bulk—the less time in the roaster, the lower the weight loss and the higher the yield. A cinnamon roast rarely appears in specialty-coffee shops, though, because it is so high in chlorogenic acid and low in body.

City and **Full-City Roast:** "City," which seems to have come into wide usage in the nineteenth century, has usually meant "dark." But as times changed, roasts got darker and new names became necessary. Today, "city" is barely darker than cinnamon, and "full-city" is used for a medium roast, more or less dark cinnamon in color and with no oil on the surface. This is the fullest development of a bean before oils appear, and the one that the East Coast chain The Coffee Connection long championed for its high-acid Central American and East African coffees. As Starbucks has been changing national tastes toward darker roasts, the full-city roast is going out of style, or acquiring a darker meaning.

Vienna Roast: The next stage—when droplets of oil just start to appear and the color is only slightly darker, handsomely speckled with dark brown spots—is usually called "Vienna." Yet more confusion: "Vienna" has also traditionally described a blend of beans taken to several different roast degrees. It is this degree of roast (whatever the name) that is taking the place of the medium, no-oil roast that was once the norm.

Italian Roast: At the next darker roast, the beans are half covered with oil droplets and the color is a uniform milk-chocolate brown verging on bittersweet chocolate. Here the names get more idiosyncratic, since everything beyond this stage was once so rare. Although people often call this darker stage an "Italian" roast, in Italy most roasts would strike today's Americans as surprisingly light. The Seattle-based coffee roaster Torrefazione Italia, where an Italian, Emanuele Bizzarri, was the founding roastmaster, breaks down roast names by Italian city. Northern cities like Milan, Venice and Perugia prefer lighter roasts; cities from Rome south to Naples and Palermo, in Sicily, prefer darker roasts.

French Roast: Rarely, if ever, do Europeans drink coffee made from roasts at the stage when oil completely covers the beans and they are the color of bittersweet chocolate. At that point, beans are heavily carbonized, and one kind of bean more or less tastes like another. Still, people persist in associating this with European sophistication and call it names like "French," "New Orleans" or plain "espresso."

Split-Second Decisions

A roaster needs the instincts of a chef and the skill of a machine operator. Even if he or she has decided in advance what the roast degree should be, real-time decisions make evenness of development something of a feat. After the first pop, when beans produce heat of their own, the roast can gallop away from a beginning roaster, even if the flame is at its lowest setting—especially if the bean is soft to begin with, for instance a low-grown Brazil.

That's why the roaster never strays far from the machine after the first pop, standing by it anxiously and constantly checking the scoop. Standard practice is to listen for that first popcorn crackle, then lower the heat.

The question is how much and for how long, since every roaster wants to control caramelization without developing a burnt taste. For a while after the first pop, a roaster might let the beans "coast," turning off the flame altogether if they seem to be going too fast—a safety measure that experienced roasters frown on. Lowering the air temperature at the very end of the roast, too, is a common trick to sweeten and smooth out the flavor of an espresso blend, which can easily become bitter if it is simply roasted to a high temperature until the beans turn blackish and oily.

But a roaster can't let the beans coast too long, to avoid the grassy tastes of a "baked" roast. In a baked roast, the outside color seems a medium brown, but so much of the acids and oils have gone up the chimney that only a flat, cardboardy taste remains. Coffee brewed from beans roasted this way is low in body, devoid of nuance and oddly shrill when hot.

Baked roasts waste time and fuel. But beans with underdeveloped, grassy flavors can also result from a roast that is performed too fast and at too high a temperature, with resultingly poor heat transfer. Shaving five minutes off an average roast time, which at normal heat can vary from nine to fourteen minutes, can greatly reduce fuel costs. Beans from a fast roast might look like any others, but a sample of the ground beans reveals the telltale difference: an under-developed interior, apparent from its much lighter color. (A too-light interior is a notorious problem with decaffeinated beans.) Other visible signs are an assortment of very dark, oily beans and light ones in the same roast, and beans "tipped" with black freckles at either end caused by escaping hot gas. Coffee brewed from beans roasted too fast, which any coffee drinker is likely to taste sooner or later, will have both burnt and grassy flavors. It lacks body and can have an unwelcome metallic overtone.

At the fateful moment the roaster decides to dispatch the roasted beans, he or she opens a half-moon-shaped door at the front of the drum. The beans cascade out with a steady, loud whoosh and tumble onto a round, shallow cooling table, attached to the drum at the operator's waist level. The metal floor of the table is perforated and attached to a ventilator; for several minutes, a rotating arm with paddles sweeps the hot beans while the ventilator sucks down air to cool them. Then they go into bins or bags.

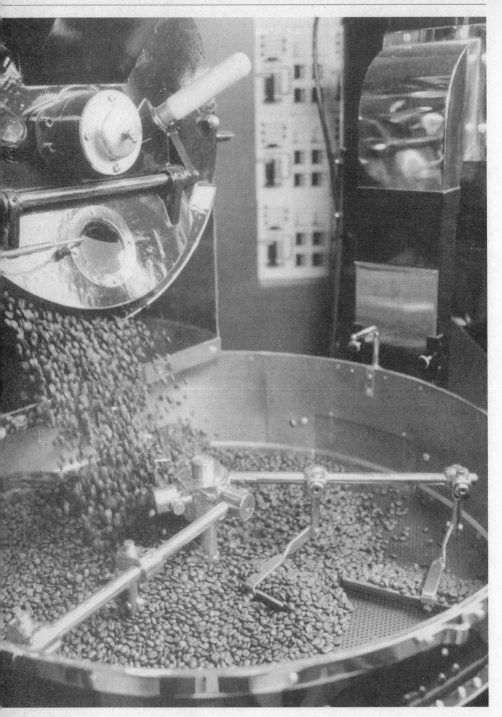

Drum coffee roaster

Big companies sometimes use "water-quenching" rather than "air-quenching," spraying beans with water to cool them. The practice is controversial. If done carefully, meaning fast and while the beans are still very hot, all the water will evaporate and cool the beans without penetrating them. Water-quenching is necessary for batches larger than the ones specialty roasters customarily use, which can't be cooled fast any other way. Sometimes, though, the water does penetrate the beans, opening their pores and allowing precious volatile flavors to escape. Roasters who favor water-quenching, including many who are very attentive to quality, say that they can judge how much water to spray on so that the beans cool properly and flavor does not suffer—an assertion that those who air-quench dismiss.

Flavored Coffees

If the beans are to be flavored—a terrible idea!—they are mixed in metal barrels with flavor extracts after they are cooled. The process is extremely simple: they're stirred around just enough to coat them with the oily, potent liquid. Many companies compete in making essences, some using synthesized and some using natural flavors. Manufacturers are now producing essences specifically for coffee beans; at one time, they simply sold flavorings that had been used for, say, ice creams and other sweets. At this stage, roasted nuts might also be added, although these are more for visual appeal than actual flavor when ground and steeped in hot water.

For a roaster, the important things to remember when adding flavor essences are to separate barrels of flavored coffees from barrels or bags of roasted unflavored coffee, because roasted beans, with their broken cell walls, easily absorb the odors around them. And cleanliness, always important, becomes even more crucial, as Paul Comey, of Green Mountain Coffee Roasters, in Vermont, points out: his company uses only stainless-steel containers for mixing and storing flavored coffees, and rinses them with very hot water every time they are emptied. If a warehouse filled with freshly roasted coffee is as intoxicating as the smell of ten thousand just-opened cans of coffee, entering a room full of different-flavored coffees—raspberry, chocolate, hazelnut, almond, mint—is like walking into a giant sundae.

High-Tech Innovations

New devices are helping the roaster produce an accurate and balanced roast. Carl Staub, a physicist in Nevada, has developed a machine he calls the Agtron, which uses near-infrared light to measure the degree of caramelization of sugars. This, he says, is the measurement that counts in determining the degree of roast. Larger companies have long used similar devices; smaller roasters are flying to Nevada to take roasting seminars. The initial results of their experiments might well be technically perfect but dull, like the wines that came from California in the 1970s, when every winemaker studied chemistry at the University of California at Davis. But more precision could help the cause of different roasts for different beans.

Roasting machines, too, are entering the high-tech era. A number of industrial companies have adopted "high-yield" machines, which cut roast times to as little as ninety seconds by using a continuous conveyor belt and blasts of superheated air. Originally developed in the 1950s, these machines, usually called "fluid-bed" roasters, keep beans aloft in a stream of hot air (thus their "fluid" movement—the process itself is very dry). The claims by manufacturers include cleaner flavor, because bits of chaff don't singe on the walls, and greater volume, since the beans puff before they lose much water. It might be that these machines, with their accurate, presettable temperature probes—impossible in conventional drum roasters—point the way toward the future of roasting, improving not only efficiency but quality too. So far, though, the majority opinion is that only the use of the hand and eye can best develop the flavor of a bean.

Sadly, technology has not come to the rescue of people who want to roast at home and who have had a few disasters with stovetop roasting. I've tried two electric home hot-air roasting machines, which fit easily onto a countertop and also have glass chambers that enable you to watch bean development. That development is agonizingly slow and invariably uneven, resulting in baked beans with hardly any body and a disappointing flatness. Also, the glass gets perilously hot, and sometimes the machine doesn't have an efficient venting mechanism for the chaff, which can fly all over the place.

Worse even than these machines (which cost $200 to $300 when I bought them around 1990), is trying to roast beans in a jury-rigged air popper meant for popcorn. Many years ago, I took the advice of two food writers I admire, who said that they wouldn't dream of drinking coffee brewed from any beans except the ones they roasted every morning in their air popper, which they had altered to be a home roaster. In following their directions, I melted the machine's plastic housing. I still find bits of chaff around the kitchen from the fountain that issued from the aluminum-foil tent they instructed me to make as a cover. Too, the heating element doesn't get hot enough to do anything but bake the beans, and you can't see the color change as you helplessly watch chaff blow everywhere.

For those who want to taste the freshest coffee possible, though, without suffering these "I Love Lucy" effects, Michael Sivetz, a producer of roasting machines in Corvallis, Oregon, manufactures a small but state-of-the-art one-ounce sample roaster that sells for $100—and a 1.25-pound roaster for $2,000 (see Sources, page 254). I haven't tried these machines, but I trust Sivetz, a seasoned engineer and advocate for better coffee.

The Right Roast

So what's the right way—the best way—to roast a bean? Not just machines but styles and philosophies vary. The disagreement over how to present a fine, high-acid coffee is a coastal battle. The East Coast camp, historically led by Joel Schapira, of the New York family that began Schapira's Coffee & Tea, and George Howell, the founder of The Coffee Connection, based in Boston, believes that roasting these coffees to anything beyond a light mahogany color with only the beginning of a gloss of oils is tantamount to a crime. This is the point at which the play of acids is at its very liveliest, when there is just enough body to keep the brewed coffee from seeming like water. Another significant adherent to this philosophy is Green Mountain Coffee Roasters.

The West Coast camp, currently led most visibly by Starbucks, favors dark roasts. The pleasing qualities of very dark roasts—heavy body, sweetness, a deep flavor that cuts through large quantities of milk and sugar— led travelers in the France of the 1950s and 1960s to associate dark roasts with sophistication. The main reason for dark roasts in France, though, is that the country traditionally bought and still buys inferior robusta beans from its former colonies.

Apart from travelers seeking to revive happy memories, real appreciation and enthusiasm for the world of coffees came to the United States only in the late 1960s, with the Dutch-born Alfred Peet, who grew up learning the coffee trade in Amsterdam. Peet brought a new idea to Berkeley, California, where he opened a shop in 1967: good arabica beans, unlike the ones used in France, roasted to a darkness typical of France. Because the quality of his beans was so much higher than that being offered by the vast majority of other roasters, he attracted a cult following.

Part of the Peet's cult included the three men who founded Starbucks, in 1971, in Seattle. One of those men, Jerry Baldwin, later bought Peet's, and with another of the founding partners, Zev Sigal, opened a new chain of shops on the East Coast named Quartermaine (since sold). The standard Peet's roast is the darkest in the country—darker than Starbucks, darker than most of what any traveler will find abroad. But it is done with remarkable finesse, and the beans are of the highest quality.

American travelers shifted loyalties from France to Italy, and in the 1980s, the mania for all things Italian sent travelers back home longing for the rich, full flavor of the espressos and cappuccinos they had tasted. This quest coincided with the arrival at Starbucks of Howard Schultz, who was brought in by the founders in 1985. Schultz soon opened hundreds of coffee shops and cafés all across the country, with a strong emphasis on espresso-based drinks.

Starbucks has brought an appreciation of the peerless power of cappuccino and espresso to the whole country. But any novice to fine coffee should get a number of catalogs and order exotic-sounding, interesting coffees and compare styles and flavors of brews. You'll embark on a lifelong quest for the newest bean from the farthest place and the best roast to bring out its aroma and depth.

4

Grinding and Storing

SOME PEOPLE say that the single most important way to improve the quality of the coffee you drink is to buy whole beans and grind them at home. But freshness comes first. The best advice is to start with good beans that have been carefully roasted within the past week. How do you know when the beans were roasted? By going to a coffee shop that tells you exactly when, and that knows how to store them so they will stay at their best. Unfortunately, few specialty shops mark each bag of coffee with the roast date—the key piece of information. Ordering by mail is usually the surest route to freshness, since specialty roasters ship beans a day or two after they are roasted. Then it's up to you to protect the beans from air, heat and light.

To ensure the best coffee from freshly roasted beans, you'll almost always want to buy whole beans and grind them just before you brew. Not only do whole beans keep better—ten days at room temperature in an opaque airtight container—but they lose aromatics much more slowly than do ground beans. A green (unroasted) bean can last for months and even years, but once beans are roasted, their natural aromatic oils break through cell walls. Your goal is to preserve the maximum possible amount of the hundreds of fragrant compounds created during roasting, because they're what give life to coffee. Grinding breaks open thousands of cells, which release aromatics into the air and take in oxygen and moisture. Air and moisture are the enemies of freshness. First the beans fade to lifelessness. Then they start going bad; air oxidizes the oils, making them taste rancid.

Grinding at home gives you the freedom to make whatever kind of coffee you fancy. In the course of a day, you might start with drip coffee, then use an inexpensive stovetop espresso machine for a midafternoon pick-me-up and steep a plunger potful of coffee after dinner. All these methods require a specific grind to come out right—more than they need any particular kind of bean or even any special roast.

In the Can

Keeping beans fresh starts with packaging and storing them right, and there's still no ideal way to arrest staling. How can you tell which beans at a gourmet shop are likely to be the freshest? Assuming that the roast date is nowhere visible on the package—unfortunatley, a good bet—the package itself can provide many clues to the condition of the beans inside.

Because every kind of package, no matter how high the technology, comes with its own tradeoffs, there's still no better way to buy beans than whole, roasted in the past week, stored away from air and light and heat, and packed simply in a greaseproof paper or plastic bag that can be tightly resealed. Anyone who doesn't live near a coffee roaster and isn't organized enough to shop by mail is fortunate that present-day packing technology has without doubt improved bean freshness.

In packaging, looks don't count. One of the least effective storage methods is the most endearing. Coffee cans are indispensable for pencils, paintbrushes, Lego pieces and bacon drippings, and they're even handy for storing whole coffee beans you've taken out of some other kind of package. But the matchless aroma of ground beans you sniff when you open the can is the whole problem: a few intoxicating moments later, precious aromatics are lost forever.

What explains this depressing phenomenon? Newly roasted beans start releasing carbon dioxide gas that is created during the final stages of roasting —a minimum of three times their volume in gas, in fact. If the freshly roasted beans are put into a can before they "degas," the escaping carbon dioxide will swell and force open the can at a weak point, generally along the seam. Even if the rupture is too small to let coffee cascade out, it certainly lets in oxygen. The same problem applies, of course, to flimsier materials like thin plastic, which could burst dramatically—an alarming scenario for a manufacturer concerned with liability.

The simplest solution for the packager is to let freshly roasted beans sit for at least twelve hours, and often for several days, until the gas dissipates. The problem is that while the carbon dioxide escapes, aromatics do too, and oxygen enters. Degassing before packaging guarantees stale coffee. Ground coffee would seem a better packaging candidate, because it degasses much faster than whole beans—a matter of hours rather than days. But the increased surface area that lets out the gas lets in staling air at the same time.

Roasting companies have found various ways around this very big problem, but the ways have mostly not involved coffee cans. Virtually all canned coffee is ground, meaning that it's bound to be well on the road to staleness by the time the buyer opens the can. The term "vacuum-packed" is misleading, because when a vacuum is used to remove air, it removes only 90 percent of it. The 2 percent oxygen left in the can is more than sufficient to stale the coffee, even if staling takes place much more slowly than it would in an open container, as Michael Sivetz of Corvallis, Oregon, a master of coffee technology, explains. And the vastly increased surface area of the ground beans means yet easier access for the oxygen.

Some high-end companies, like illycaffè, a top-of-the-line Italian es-presso roaster, do put whole roasted rather than ground beans into cans, and take the expensive step of substituting for the remaining oxygen an inert gas, such as nitrogen or, more commonly, carbon dioxide. Illy says that it inserts carbon dioxide under pressure, which forces the oils back into the beans, resulting in evenly flavored, mellow coffee. Critics complain that this homogenizes the taste, but the removal of oxygen does help keep the beans fresher.

Coffee cans—the kind with keys to open them—are already bought and sold by collectors who consult books for rarity and current prices. Coffee cans never existed in many countries, and they hardly exist anymore in oth-ers. Is this because manufacturers found a better way to maintain freshness? No. They found a cheaper way.

Brick Packs and Pillow Packs

The less expensive method is, in effect, to shrink-wrap the beans, usually ground, in "brick packs"—thick plastic bags that hug the pebbled outline of whole beans or the gritty surface of ground coffee and relax as soon as they are cut open. Brick packs, which were developed in Germany in the 1950s but only decades later came into wide use in the United States, save both the price of metal and a good deal of storage space. They don't deliver coffee much superior to what comes out of a can, though. For one thing, the coffee is also degassed and put under a vacuum before being packaged. And the bags are inconvenient. They aren't resealable, the way cans are, so the easi-est way to store what remains is just to let the open bag sit on the counter—about as bad a way as there is to keep coffee. A rubber band will help some, but you really should transfer the contents of the opened bag to an opaque airtight container.

An obvious solution to the packaging problem is to put coffee straight from the roasting machine into a container that will let out gas. For years, roasters have supplied ground coffee to commercial customers in "pillow packs"—soft packages usually about 5 inches square, which hold enough coffee to brew one pot. They are flushed with an inert gas and can contain pinprick holes to allow carbon dioxide to escape. So far, so good: the inert gas means that the package starts out with no oxygen inside, and for a few days, the pressure of the escaping gas prevents any new oxygen from entering. After a few days, though, this is a very poor method: the gas that needed to get out is gone, and oxygen is free to enter through the tiny holes (not every packager includes these). The method is still common, and it can be easily defended, say, in the case of a large-volume restaurant or hotel that receives frequent deliveries of fresh coffee from a local roaster. These, in fact, are the only customers for pillow packs—you won't find them in specialty shops or supermarkets.

Having It Both Ways: Valve-Lock Bags

Only in the 1960s did someone come up with a way both to allow carbon dioxide to escape and to prevent oxygen from entering. This was the long-awaited breakthrough—the first package of real use to the home consumer and the high-quality roaster. The invention, the work of an Italian engineer named Luigi Goglio, is a one-way valve about the shape of a nickel, with a little hole in the middle. The valve is mounted nearly invisibly into laminated plastic, which is cut and folded into a bag. Roasted beans, whole or ground, can be put into valve-lock bags as soon as they are cool. The bags aren't as neatly shaped as brick packs and are often puffy. Unlike brick packs, which should be taut, valve-lock bags are supposed to be soft. To tell if a bag has a valve, run your finger across the surface. The valve is usually on the front, near the top; you can feel the small, round disc, and if you hold the pinprick-sized hole to your nose, you can smell the beans.

Valve-lock bags are by far the best way to package coffee that must be stored for more than, say, a week after roasting before the customer goes home with it. But they aren't ideal. Many roasters subject the coffee to a vacuum before packing it into the bag, which removes some aromatics; others instead flush the bags with nitrogen. Some of the aroma that remains escapes as the beans degas and as customers eagerly press and sniff the bags. The bags won't give coffee an infinite shelf life, either. Careful roasters claim that coffee from a valve-lock bag is undrinkable after four months, but most roasters put far more optimistic shelf-life dates on them. Because they cost a good deal more than other packaging material and do not stack on pallets as easily as brick packs or cans, valve-lock bags are likely to remain the province of the specialty roaster.

Too, all the benefits of valves cease as soon as the package is opened. Make sure before you buy a valve-lock bag of coffee that the top of the package is heat-sealed. I've visited shops that took out half the beans in a one-pound package, taped the top shut, then put it back on the shelf. As soon as you break the seal at home, you'll need the right container for storing the remaining coffee.

Storage Fundamentals

Even if you go straight to a store that stocks freshly roasted whole beans, you can't be sure that the beans have been stored impeccably. Good specialty stores keep beans in opaque bins, often in garbage bags inside the bins or barrels. Garbage bags are ugly, to be sure, but they are actually a fine way to make sure that the beans stay away from light, heat and moisture—and that their oils won't soak into the wood if the bins are wooden, and go rancid. Often you'll see beans in glass jars or Lucite bins, which admit constant light and are rarely cleaned out between loads.

Lucite bins, the commonest supermarket storage containers, are especially hard to keep clean, because oils from the beans easily and invisibly build up and turn rancid. It's doubtful that many markets regularly wash out their Lucite bins with hot water and dry them thoroughly. Keeping flavored beans close to unflavored ones is also dangerous, because aromas from the flavored beans can so easily penetrate the unflavored ones.

The best way to store beans, ground or whole, is to empty them into an opaque, airtight canister of a size just big enough so that there is as little air at the top as possible. This is easier at home than in a supermarket. Catalogs and stores offer ceramic canisters, used also for other dry goods like pasta and rice, with metal rings that latch shut. (The mail-order company Gevalia sells nice ones and occasionally features them as gifts with orders.) If you keep only one or two kinds of beans around and keep the canister full, these will serve you well.

If you like to try different blends and have little ends of bags you want to keep as fresh as possible (as is always the case in my kitchen), you might go to a kitchen-supply shop to find plastic tubs with tight-fitting lids, usually sold as flour or sugar canisters. I stuff half-empty bags of beans, held shut with an elastic band, into one of these tubs, and try to remember when I bought each bag so that I can use up the beans in order; if you're organized, label the bags by kind of bean and date.

Most bags aren't easily resealed, which is why I resort to elastic bands. Some bags have flexible wire-clamp closures attached across the top. Tin ties, as they are called in the trade, seem to fall off the first time you use them; the glue never sticks right, especially if the bag is plastic. Paper bags lined with a grease-proof coating, still the norm among specialty roasters, are a decent way to keep coffee, but once you get the beans home from the store, it's better to store them in a tightly sealed ceramic or plastic container.

The Freezer Controversy

I've never been fully happy with either refrigerating or freezing coffee. Certainly, refrigeration is a bad idea. If stored in a refrigerator, beans can absorb odors; this is particularly a problem with ground coffee, which is so absorbent that it used to be recommended as a refrigerator freshener. The freezer is a better option, one I have recently been persuaded to rethink by Michael Sivetz, who in the 1950s conducted studies on storing coffee. He concluded that freezing removed fewer aromatics than other forms of storage. Still, the freezer is controversial. Ground coffee can absorb freezer odors. The oils in beans, especially apparent in a dark roast, congeal when frozen, and some people claim that they never return to their original consistency, harming the body of the brewed coffee, particularly espresso.

My opinion is that refrigeration virtually guarantees off flavors in ground or whole beans, and that coffee never tastes quite the same after it has been frozen—even if freezing is far better than refrigerating. But if you can't use up your beans within two weeks or so, settle for putting them into the freezer, whole and tightly sealed, in either a glass jar or plastic container.

Getting the Right Grind

The difficulties of packaging and storing ground beans to retain maximum freshness have led to the unbreakable rule that you should always grind beans at home just before brewing. I think the rule is breakable in the case of espresso, because pump espresso machines—the kind that achieve the proper degree of pressure—require a uniform, fine grind in order for the liquid to have *crema*, or golden foam, floating atop it, and inexpensive grinders can't reliably produce such a fine grind. For regular forms of brewing, though, like drip and plunger pot, the right grind makes all the difference to a good cup—and home grinders can achieve it.

The right grind matters so much because each brewing method has its ideal time to achieve the correct extraction, or amount of soluble solids that pass from beans to water. "Extraction of soluble solids" sounds like something from a chemistry lab, and it is, but it's the measure of whether a brewing method has the correct amount of body and flavor. (See Chapter Five, "Brewing," for a longer discussion of extraction and the right amount of coffee to water, which is also crucial.)

The shorter the brewing time, the finer the grind must be, for a quick and thorough extraction: espresso, which has a brewing time of half a minute or less, requires a very fine grind. The longer the brewing time, the coarser the grind should be, to avoid overextraction of undesirable substances: plunger-pot coffee—in which coffee grounds steep in water, the way tea leaves do, for a full five or six minutes—requires a very coarse grind.

Cool Precision: The Burr Mill

Almost everyone who grinds coffee at home owns a propeller grinder with a single two-sided blade that spins around. Propeller grinders are small, most of them cost between $15 and $30, and they take up little counter space. But they aren't very efficient. The kind everyone should own instead is a coffee mill, also called a burr mill, whose two shredding discs, or burrs, are grooved and can be adjusted to be closer or farther apart depending on how fine or coarse a grind is necessary. A burr mill is an essential investment—much more essential than an electric brewer, for instance. Cheaper and equally good methods for brewing coffee are available, but there's no substitute for a grinder that will produce the same result time after time and give you a superior cup of coffee.

The notched metal discs of the coffee mill revolve against each other and shred the beans a few at a time. This is the same principle by which people have ground wheat and other grains for millennia, using millstones,

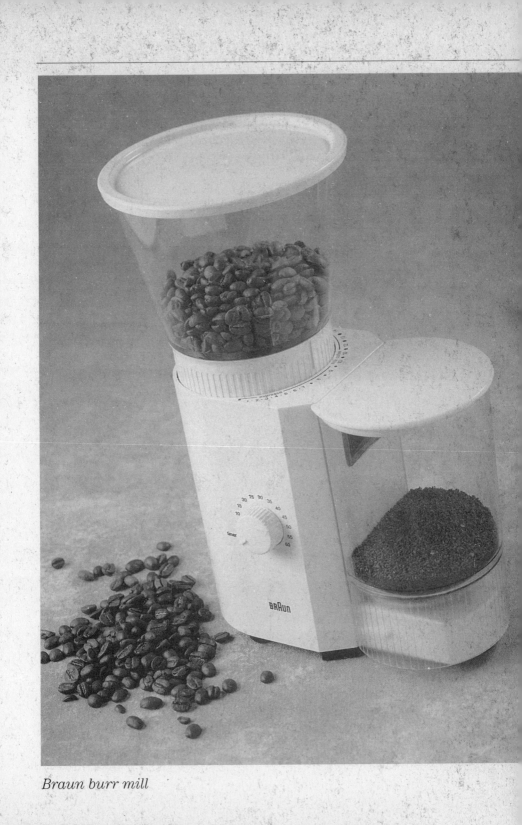

Braun burr mill

which were once traditional for coffee merchants too. Home grinding meant using a mortar and pestle—an essential prop for the Middle Eastern ritual of preparing coffee, which involved roasting, crushing and boiling coffee while honored guests looked on. Apart from the elbow grease required, a mortar and pestle is a poor way to grind beans. They heat up during the crushing, releasing aromatics that should go into the hot water during brewing and not into the air.

Cool, precise tearing apart is what's called for. Large manufacturers use roller mills that cut the beans apart powerfully and fast, so fast that the beans don't heat up. Sometimes the rollers themselves are cold, chilled internally by cold water as an extra precaution against heating the beans.

The closest you can come to this icy precision at home is with the burr mill. The Solis Maestro, a current favorite for its sleek design, accuracy and ease of use, costs about $125; Bodum's burr mill costs about $50, and Braun's model costs about $60. Home burr mills work much more slowly than propeller grinders. Beans must pass between the whirling plates at a fixed rate, and the more beans, the longer it takes. But you can grind as much or as little as you like and get a reliably consistent result. Just put the beans into the hopper, set a knob to how coarse or fine you want the grind, and turn on the machine. The switches on several machines automatically shut off after a time determined by how far you turn the dial.

No home burr mill is perfect, the way professional models, which after all cost many hundreds and even thousands of dollars, often are. But the relative precision they offer and the enormous gain in freshness make them preferable. Imperfections include the noise home mills make: it will drown out just about any radio and certainly any conversation. The wait can seem endless. And it's impossible to extract every last particle from the containers of home mills without getting ground coffee on the counter and your hands.

Some mills excel at coarser grinds, for filter and plunger-pot coffee, and others at finer grinds. The Bunn, for example, a boxy machine with a powerful motor, is excellent on all grinds in the coarse range, from campfire, or hobo, coffee (the coarsest—little rocks) to plunger pot to paper filter. Even though it's the best of the commonly available mills I've tried, it doesn't do as well on the finer range for stovetop espresso and electric espresso machines. Braun's burr mill, by contrast, is very good for fine grinds but not as good for coarse.

Of course, there are always the hand-cranked grinders of yore, the ones that turn up at flea markets and get converted to lamps. These are burr mills, too, and they offer all the advantages of precise grinding—plus the advantage of a workout, if you're so inclined. They come in several styles: those that sit on a counter, with the crank on top; those that clamp onto the edge of the counter, with the crank on the side, which allows a more natural arm movement; and those that are mounted on the wall, just like coffee grinders in folklife museums. All these grinders have adjustable burrs that produce consistent results; the best-known manufacturer is Zassenhaus. Good ones are just as expensive as their electric descendants, though, and it takes forever to get enough ground coffee for a decent-sized pot. If you loathe electricity and seek serious forearm toning, you might want to buy one.

At the other end of the gaddget spectrum are the burr mills that come with some models of espresso machines—the most expensive models. These grind precisely, finely and quickly enough to meet the demands of any espresso machine, home or professional, and of course they can be set to grind coffee for most other brewing methods, although their range is mostly in fine grinds. The drawback is price. Even sold separately from the espresso machine, as they sometimes are, they usually start at $150.

Electric burr mills usually come with guides saying which setting to use for the brewing method you want. Don't assume they will be accurate. The quickest way around this problem is to check a home-ground sample against a sample of ground coffee from an experienced coffee shop (see page 64).

Professional grinders at local supermarkets for public use—even my 7-Eleven has one—are usually inaccurate, because they suffer from heavy and often careless use, and the grinding plates rarely receive the regular calibration they need. (This alignment problem doesn't seem to affect home burr mills, perhaps because the plates are so much smaller.) You can assume that the grind will be one or two settings coarser than the little pictures on the dial say it is. Before you begin, always run a few fresh beans through, on the assumption that a bit of noxious flavored coffee remains from the previous customer. Then grind a few beans at a time, testing the grind by rubbing it between your fingers to see if it matches the feeling you remember from the samples you got at a reliable coffee shop.

The Propeller Grinder

Unfortunately, propeller grinders fall closer to the brute force of mortar and pestle than to the ripping precision of roller mills. The disadvantages become clear if you look at coffee from a propeller grinder through a magnifying glass and compare it to coffee from a decent burr mill. The burrs produce dark brown, dry, separate granules, as neatly shaped and distinct as salt crystals. The surface of granules from a propeller grinder is dull and oily; the particles clump in a rocky, greasy way recognizable to any cook who has put nuts into a food processor hoping for nut flour for a cake and ended up with chunky nut butter instead. Worse, the granules produced by a propeller grinder vary greatly in size, from the fine powder beneath the blade at the bottom of the chamber to the coarser pieces at the top. This powder, or "fines," can slow the passage of water through coffee in a filter, causing bitter and sour substances to enter the brew.

Because so many people own propeller grinders, here are some hints for getting the best results from them. It's better to grind a bit coarse to avoid the problem of fines clouding your brew. Aim for ten-second bursts: don't whir beans for more than thirty seconds, which will overheat them badly. Try not to grind more than 4 scoops (½ cup) at a time, because the chamber is rarely big enough to do a decent job on more than that; some models can handle 6 scoops. Lift the machine off the counter and shake it while it grinds, as if it had martinis inside. Do a little dance to keep the beans circulating as much and as evenly as possible around the blade. To remove the ground beans easily, turn the grinder upside down and rap it sharply on a table—this is an emphatic activity. Then carefully lift out the inverted base of the grinder. (For timing recommendations, see page 65.)

You can make up for some of the deficiencies of propeller grinders by keeping them whistle-clean. Unplug them first, of course. At the minimum, wipe out the grinding chamber with a damp paper towel or sponge after each use, and wash the plastic top in hot water. This procedure won't be sufficient if you buy flavored coffees, though, because yesterday's raspberry decaf will mix with the day before's streusel coffee cake and today's Swiss chocolate almond. The more scrupulous way to clean a propeller grinder is to put in two or three tablespoons of sugar and whir it for twenty or thirty seconds; wipe out the chamber and wash the lid. This step is essential if you ever use the

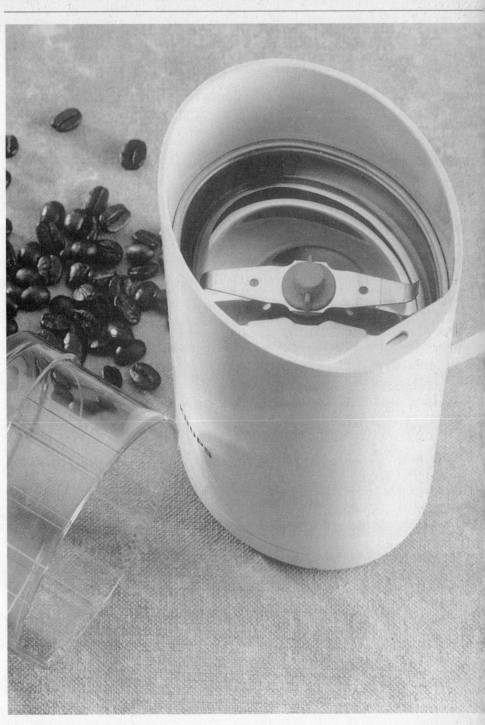

Krups propeller mill

GRINDING AT A GLANCE

The best way to know whether you're using the right grind is to go to a specialty-coffee shop and ask for a sample. To gauge the feel and look, rub it between your fingers and put some ground coffee on a white surface and poke it around. Powder, or fines, will stay on your fingers; grit will fall off. Then grind a few beans in your home machine to reproduce the look and feel of the sample.

If you have a propeller grinder, grind no more than 4 scoops (½ cup) at a time, using short bursts of ten to twenty seconds and shaking the grinder to keep the beans in motion.

Set the dial of a burr mill to the setting the manufacturer recommends for your brewing method and adjust up or down until you match the sample from the shop.

Middle Eastern or Turkish: The finest of all, as soft and fine as all-purpose white flour, with the feel of flannel. This is best left to a shop: propeller grinders will overheat the beans while trying to achieve this, and home burr mills rarely grind finely enough.

Electric pump espresso: Not as soft as flour between the fingers but still very fine, between flour and table salt. You're best off getting this grind from a specialty-coffee shop or even prepackaged, because electric pump machines require consistent and fine grinds to make good espresso. But home burr mills can achieve them, especially the more expensive ones.

Stovetop espresso, or moka: A medium to fine grit, like fine sand.

Paper-filter drip: For wedge-shaped filters, medium grit, with no powder, or fines, which will clog the filter and slow brewing. For flat-bottomed "cupcake" filters, less fine—a bit coarser than granulated sugar.

Metal-filter drip, or flip-drip (napoletana): Medium to coarse grit, with no powder, which can travel through the pores of the metal and cause sediment in the brewed coffee. Check your fingers: they should be clean.

Vacuum pot: Medium grit, with little powder.

Plunger pot, or French press: Coarse flakes, like bread crumbs or cornmeal. Feels like coarse sandpaper.

Open pot, or cowboy or hobo: Coarse, cracked beans, like cracked black pepper, with a wide range of particle sizes.

Timing the Propeller Grinder

It's hard to give exact timings for the propeller, because both the machines and the people operating them vary so much. But here are recommendations from Bruce Mullins, a longtime roaster and seller of coffee equipment in Portland, Oregon. These recommendations are for a full grinder: shave off a few seconds for fewer than 4 scoops.

Plunger Pot	10 seconds
Manual or Electric Drip:	
Flat-bottomed paper filters	13 seconds
Wedge-shaped gold filters	13 seconds
Wedge-shaped paper filters	16 seconds

grinder for spices, although it's a better idea to keep a separate grinder for that purpose. Conscientious gourmet shops use different grinders for flavored coffees, knowing how persistent the residues of extracts can be.

There's little point in recommending one propeller grinder over another, because the differences are small. If you're looking for consistent and accurate grinds, nothing has the edge over a burr mill. It will remove needless guesswork from coffee making, and will make brewing the satisfying morning ritual it should be.

5 | Brewing

JUST AS THERE IS NO BEST COFFEE BEAN, there is no best way to brew coffee. But some ways are better than others, and a few simple steps can vastly improve your everyday brew. Here are the first: be careful about freshness, use the right grind, and don't skimp on the scoops. One change of habit will improve your life drastically: never, ever leave coffee on a burner.

Now that espresso is so popular, people are looking for coffee more potent than what they grew up drinking. Only the high pressure of an espresso machine will produce espresso's uniquely thick texture, but there are ways to beef up anemic home brews. Using the correct amount of coffee will give you a denser-textured, fuller-flavored cup than you're probably used to, and so will a less obvious trick: substituting a metal filter for a paper one.

Brewing coffee right reveals the full spectrum of aromas and flavors in your beans—aromas and flavors you might have been missing. Besides, espresso is over in a few power-packed swallows. Brewed coffee keeps you company.

A Satisfying Extraction

How do you get the very best cup of coffee you can at home? The ideal is a liquid with just the right extraction of coffee solids for a textured, deeply flavored brew—but not too many solids, which would turn the liquid bitter, cardboard-flavored or both. The extraction rate is the percentage of soluble solids—all the different substances that can be tasted—that go from the beans into your brew. The extraction rate may sound needlessly technical, but it's the yardstick experts use to judge how good a brewing machine or method is, and it's central to explaining why a cup of coffee is satisfying or disappointing. And you can adopt your own brewing habits to achieve the ideal rate.

At first glance, squeezing absolutely everything out of a coffee bean might seem a good idea. Why waste a bit of what gives coffee its flavor and body? Coffee people do dismiss sour, thin, grassy coffee as "underextracted," meaning that not enough soluble solids came out. But efficiency is good only up to a point. The same people call harshly potent coffee "overextracted," meaning that too many soluble solids came out.

The extraction rate depends on how hot the water is, how long the ground coffee remains in contact with the water, and how fine or coarse the grind is. The ideal water temperature is about 195 to 205 degrees F—not a rolling boil, which will extract bitter substances you don't want to taste. Long contact time is the surest way to overextract coffee: no brewing with hot water should go on longer than eight minutes. The rate is much faster for finely ground beans, with their hundreds of thousands of broken cells and exponentially increased surface area, than for coarsely ground beans.

Roasted coffee beans contain about 30 percent soluble solids, and most experts put the ideal extraction rate at 18 to 22 percent. This doesn't mean that your cup will be 22 percent solids. That would be coffee porridge. It means that 22 percent of what can come out of the beans actually does. The dissolved solids account for only between 1 and 2 percent of the brewed liquid. Coffee itself, then, is only a small part of what you drink. The big part is water.

The Main Ingredient — Water

A cup of coffee is more than 98 percent water. Think a minute. Do you like the taste of your tap water? Is it what you put in a pitcher to stay cold in the refrigerator? I know people who use bottled water for their coffee, but it seems a bit let-'em-eat-cake to me, unless the kitchen is big enough for a home water cooler and it's easy to lay in a large supply. Don't use distilled water, the kind for steam irons or contact lenses: the absence of mineral content, which keeps both irons and lenses clean, means a drink with no interest at all. Have you tasted distilled water? It's like drinking air.

Unpleasant tastes in tap water do show up in coffee, so it would be foolish to ignore the matter. "Hard" water contains alkalines, or dissolved base minerals, which can react with and neutralize the precious flavor-giving acids in coffee. Too, at high levels, the mineral salts in hard water can interfere with extraction. Even less desirable is softened water, whose phosphates and other agents can impart a soapy taste.

The way to remove off flavors like chlorine from water is with a filter, either the kind that screws onto your tap or a filter holder set into a pitcher, a method I find simple and inexpensive. Filtration pitchers, the most common manufacturer of which is Brita, come in various sizes and offer a quick and easy way to improve your drinking water. The standard filter material is charcoal; be sure to buy replacement filters when you buy the pitcher.

Cold tap water is thought to be fresher than warm because it hasn't been sitting around in a boiler or a pipe for a while, picking up off tastes from sediment or rust. Nevertheless, brewing will be that much faster if you start with hot water (electric drip machines work better with cold). But will it change the flavor? Try drinking some hot water from the tap, waiting for it to cool to judge it fairly against cool tap water.

Another reason cited for using cold water is that it contains more oxygen, which is supposed to mean brisker, livelier flavor. I've never found anyone to back up this rule with scientific evidence: according to the head of the research and test unit of the International Coffee Organization, in London, a high oxygen content in water makes no difference. Many people insist that oxygenated water does taste better, though; to judge for yourself, leave a glassful out overnight, allowing the oxygen to dissipate, to see how it tastes against freshly drawn water.

Convenience Brewing

The best brewing method is one convenient enough for you to use all the time. The goal in choosing, I think, should be to eliminate the filters that screen out both coffee oils and the colloids they form. Oils? Colloids? Have we turned to a discussion of toxic waste? No. These are both compounds you want to retain.

Coffee oil is where the "mouthfeel" is. Don't be concerned about the idea of oil in your cup: the amount is tiny, so calories are negligible. And colloids —the suspended particles of coffee solids that are too large to dissolve fully but small enough to pass through a metal filter—give coffee its texture.

Steeping ground coffee in hot water, like tea, will supply the most colloids and thus the most body—the way open-pot coffee is made, and the way professionals "cup" coffees. The most familiar home infusion method is the plunger pot, also called the French press or, after a popular French manufacturer, the Melior. In this method, after ground coffee steeps in hot water for a few minutes, you plunge a finely perforated screen down through the liquid to separate grounds from brewed coffee. Many coffee connoisseurs swear by the plunger pot, which, however simple in concept, is not the simplest in practice.

Then there is the vacuum pot, a mad-scientist contraption with double glass globes in which water comes to a boil in the bottom globe, is forced up into the second where it mixes with ground coffee, and is pulled back to the bottom, passing through a filter on the way down. A vacuum pot produces the compact disc of coffees: nothing interferes with your experience of the flavor. Vacuum pots require no power other than heat for the water, but they do require both time and cleanup.

The two extremes of filtered coffee, then, are thick coffee from a plunger pot and sediment-free liquid from a vacuum pot. My favorite brewing method is between the two, and the commonest—drip. Drip is pretty basic:

pour hot water over ground coffee in a filter. The beans must be fresh, of course, and ground to the correct fineness. And you need to use enough.

The right amount trips up nearly everyone. Big commercial roasters have for years made misleading promises that with *their* coffee you can get by using less than you actually need. Many brewing-machine manufacturers have acquired the nasty habit of supplying a scoop half the right size, to make you think you'll waste less coffee using their machines. The right-size scoop holds 2 tablespoons, or ⅛ cup of ground or whole-bean coffee. So many scoops today are half-size that it's a good idea to pour a tablespoon of water into the scoop to measure its capacity: you'll likely find that it holds only a tablespoon.

Using enough coffee to water will make an enormous difference, especially to those who have been mistaking a half-size for a full-size scoop. Happily, the measurements of whole beans and ground coffee are, for practical purposes, equal. The golden rule of brewing has traditionally been to use 1 standard coffee scoop (holding 2 tablespoons) or 2 half-size scoops to 6 ounces of water. My own preferred ratios are more generous with coffee, especially when using small amounts (see Brewing Proportions, page 93). If you prefer weaker coffee, it will taste better if you make it full strength and then dilute it with hot water or milk.

The four pieces of equipment I find essential for superb drip coffee are a grinder, a measuring cup, a gold-washed metal filter and a thermal carafe. I'm not bothering to mention the kettle, and I'm deliberately leaving out an electric drip machine, which hogs counter space and brews coffee no better, and often worse, than a simple manual method.

Do I think you'll take my advice and throw out your machine? No. So I'll begin by telling you how to improve coffee brewed in an electric drip machine. Once you get it to perform as best it can, you will at least be guaranteed consistent results. We'll assume that you've bought a charcoal filter if you don't like the taste of your tap water, and that you have a clean grinder and fresh beans at the ready.

Filters: The Value of Gold

The big question is, paper or metal filters? Paper traps texture-giving colloids; metal filters let them through. If you can't stand even a bit of sediment at the bottom of your cup, you'll want to use paper. I like metal better. I respect those who disagree, for example Kevin Knox, a founding roaster and buyer of Allegro Coffee Company, who prefers the clarity of paper-filtered coffee. He says it keeps longer too. The colloids that remain in coffee brewed through a gold filter or in a plunger pot, he says, keep on brewing as the coffee sits, eventually imparting the unpleasant flavors of overextraction. But you shouldn't try to hold brewed coffee more than forty minutes anyway.

Paper filters are certainly easier and cleaner. Consumers in recent years grew wary of using them, because of concern about dioxins, which are thought to be particularly potent carcinogens and which form during paper bleaching. Beginning in 1985, environmentalists targeted paper manufacturers that used the chlorine bleaching process, and there was a brief period of public alarm over possible dioxin residues in coffee brewed through filter paper. In the end, neither the Environmental Protection Agency nor the Food and Drug Administration, which had given conflicting risk estimates of exposure to dioxin, thought the risk from coffee filters to be significant.

The environmental issue of releasing dioxins into streams and air did not disappear, though, and environment-minded consumers turned to unbleached filters. True unbleached paper, like unbleached cotton, is beige, not brown; sometimes manufacturers add brown coloring to paper to convince consumers that it's really unbleached. Unbleached filters in turn raised concerns over possible health problems from resins and other impurities that remain in unprocessed paper. Far worse for coffee lovers, these impurities can make coffee taste like glue or tar. Unbleached filters are today washed more carefully than they once were, so there is less danger that off flavors will appear in coffee made with them.

The solution is "oxygen-bleached" filters, which were first sold to home consumers by Green Mountain Coffee Roasters in Vermont, and are today standard for commercial filter brewers. Oxygen bleaching usually involves the final bleaching of paper with chlorine dioxide, a compound of chlorine that does not create dioxin residues. If you are concerned about chemicals or off flavors and prefer the convenience of paper, oxygen-bleached filters are the best choice. They give you white paper without endangering the environment —or at least while endangering it less—and reduce health risks from virtually nil to nil.

With any paper filter, you can take the precaution of pouring hot water through the empty filter, to rinse it, before putting in the ground coffee. (Aim the water right for the bottom, or one side of the filter might well fold and stick to the other half.) Avoid storing paper filters in a cabinet with curry or cayenne or other strong-flavored spices, because filters will absorb the odors of whatever they're near.

Anyone especially concerned about the environment can use cloth filters, which fit into filter holders in place of paper or metal. They're hard to keep clean. Oils collect in cloth filters and go rancid. The cloth turns gray-brown after the first use and never returns to white unless you bleach it, which of course will leave an unwelcome taste in your coffee. An old way to keep cloth filters fresh is to store them in a jar of water after rinsing them; remember to change the water fairly frequently.

Many people assume that the only thing to do if you run out of paper filters is to use paper towels. This is a very bad idea. Water races through the paper, which often tears, and the coffee is unbearably weak and likely to have terrible tastes from bleaches, resins and inks. (Paper bags would be a better idea than paper towels—at least they slow down the water—if most of them didn't have such high resin contents.)

The main argument in favor of paper filters is cleanup: with one rap, you dump them along with the spent grounds into the wastebasket or the compost pail. Gold filters must be washed after every use. They can go into the dishwasher, although after a couple of years, the plating will begin to wear away and you'll have to buy a new one.

Gold filters come in different sizes and cost around $15, and on some electric drip machines they are standard issue. To my mind, they more than repay the investment and minor maintenance by dramatically improving taste and saving money spent on paper filters. You'll also help the cause of environmental conservation, however humbly.

Electric Drip Machines: What Matters Most

I was once told on good authority that most brands of electric drip machines are manufactured by the same group of factories around Hong Kong, and companies merely select from a book of various features or specify their own fillips here or there. I've since learned that the authority wasn't so good, and that many countries produce the machines. Still, I have found that specific brands rarely matter. What matters is wattage.

You're better off buying a large and high-end brewer, not because you should always be ready to serve a crowd but because expensive machines are usually more powerful. The important feature is one you can't see—the heater. Most machines don't heat brewing water quickly or evenly enough, so brewing cycles start too cold and take too long. The right water temperature, somewhere between 195 and 205 degrees F, and brewing-cycle time, ideally four to six minutes, will extract the desired amount of soluble substances, 18 to 22 percent. The lower temperature of less-powerful machines results in underextraction of the substances you want to taste. Many sleek European brewers are the worst offenders, requiring a sluggish ten to twelve minutes to brew ten cups—twice as much time as they should. The power they have is typically hogged by a burner, which shouldn't even be part of the machine.

The only clue a consumer has to temperature or time is the wattage. The higher it is, and thus the more powerful the heater, the better the coffee. A desirable rating is over 1,000 watts, but most home machines average around 850 watts. American machines like Mr. Coffee, the first electric drip machine to become popular in U.S. households, and now Cuisinart, Capresso, Salton and Philips among others, frequently offer high wattages.

The example to follow is set by a Dutch company, Technivorm, which manufactures electric drip brewers that adhere to the strict standards set some years ago by the Coffee Brewing Center, a now-defunct branch of the International Coffee Organization. Its machines feature powerful heaters, fast brew cycles and also the utopian innovation of thermal carafes; unfortunately, they cost about $180 and are hard to find (see Sources, page 253).

A good compromise for far less money is the Bunn Home Brewer, which uses a fast and hot cycle and the efficient flat-basket filter, called a "cupcake" filter in the trade, which requires wavy-sided filter paper. This shape, familiar from Mr. Coffee and all its imitators, by now looks clunky, because the better-looking European machines use the wedge. But professionals prefer it, saying that water saturates the ground coffee better and more evenly.

High-end machines often come freighted with useless or downright bad features. Particularly destructive is the brew-interrupt feature, which keeps brewed coffee from dripping into the carafe and enables impatient people to yank out the carafe before the brew cycle is over and pour themselves a cup of coffee. This throws off the balance of the whole batch. The first two or three cups are far stronger than the rest, because the first 60 percent of the water extracts 80 to 85 percent of the soluble solids. It might sound as though the early bird gets the best coffee, but anyone will likely find the first few cups bitter, and the poor souls who happen on the machine afterward will wonder why the coffee is so weak. (Experienced coffee makers use the brew-interrupt feature to steep the ground coffee with water in the filter for a minute or so at the beginning of the brew cycle with the carafe removed, in order to imitate the plunger pot. But this is tricky retooling. If you want this flavor and feel, you'll be safer using a plunger pot.)

Some expensive machines also offer a brew-ahead programming feature that allows you to begin brewing at a fixed time—typically, the minute the alarm rings. Purists argue that ground coffee will stale as it sits around and water will lose oxygen. But in the closed chamber of the filter basket, the ground coffee won't lose much more flavor than in a container with a better seal, and the water won't suffer that much either. If you can figure out how to set the timer, don't be shy about using it.

A gadget I find useless is a brewer that incorporates a grinder for all-in-one brewing. The built-in propeller grinders are imprecise, and the particle size varies tremendously, with fine particles that can clog the filter mixed with coarse shards that allow water to zip through. Too, it is inconvenient to clean out the grinder. These machines have a zany charm, but they're not assets to coffee lovers.

Neither are closed filter holders in place of holders you can open easily. The closed system is supposed to keep in aroma and steam, locking the flavors right into the brewed coffee. But a coffee meddler would much rather be able to swing out the filter holder in order to check the distribution of water in the ground coffee and stir it up if there are dry patches.

The two most useful features of high-priced machines involve water. One is a filter in the reservoir (be sure to find out where to get replacement cartridges when you buy such a machine). The other is a calcium sensor that lights when too much lime has built up in the machine.

Calcification is a problem in any coffee maker, and every machine should be cleaned regularly—say once a month. Mineral scaling can clog the tubes and thus undesirably extend brewing time. Several powders on the market clean and decalcify brewers (one, Better Brew, comes in a plastic packet and is sold in many specialty-coffee stores; see Sources, page 254). The process is simple: dissolve the contents of one packet in a carafe of water and run the brew cycle. You can also use a solution of 1 part white vinegar to 3 parts water. In either case, you'll have to run clear water through the brewer three to five times after you clean it; taste some water from the last cycle to be sure you don't need to run another one.

This cleaning will also remove sediment and built-up coffee oil, which collects in the plastic filter holder and in the carafe. Both these parts should also be scrubbed after every pot of coffee you brew. If you have a dishwasher, this is no problem—but you should still buy a cleaner for the machine, since the reservoir and the tubes need to be decalcified. Some people claim that dishwashing liquid leaves a funny taste. I prefer a clean machine to one with tan and brown streaks. One answer is to scrub the filter holder and carafe in hot water after every use, and in soapy water once a week or so. Another is to use instead of soap a paste of baking soda and water, which will not leave any off flavors.

The right amount of ground coffee can easily overfill the basket of an electric brewer and make it run over during the brew cycle, especially if you're brewing a full pot. In theory, there should be the same amount of headroom as ground coffee in a filter basket; combined with water, the ground coffee will nearly double in volume. Baskets on electric brewers, though, are seldom designed to leave this much room, especially wedge-shaped ones; cupcake filters allow more headroom.

Overflow is particularly likely when you use freshly roasted and ground beans: the high content of carbon dioxide bubbles through the water during brewing. A silty brown pool can seep out around the carafe—or worse, into the carafe itself. If you know that the beans have been roasted within the past three days, don't try making more than half a pot at a time, unless you think to grind the beans the night before or long enough in advance to let them degas. An excellent tip to prevent overflow comes from Jerry Baldwin, a founder of Starbucks and currently the head of Peet's: put all the coffee and half the water into the machine, and at the end of the brewing, pour the remaining amount of water (hot, of course) directly into the carafe.

As with every brewing method, grind matters. The uneven grind produced by propeller grinders intensifies the problem of overflow: even a grind that looks medium to coarse, the right kind for an electric drip machine, may have enough fines to clog the filter. Some ground coffee will remain untouched, because water will find ways around clumps of fine-ground coffee. A medium-coarse grind is safer than a fine grind in an electric drip machine, whether you use a paper or metal filter. (Also, with very fresh beans, the coarser the grind the less likely the filter is to overflow.) If you do experience an overflow, be sure after you mop up that the small holes at the base of the filter basket are still clear.

It's a good rule to empty the filter basket as soon as the coffee is brewed, to get fresh coffee away from spent coffee grounds. Condensed steam can pass again through the spent grounds and drip back into the good coffee. Worse yet is repouring brewed coffee through spent grounds because it isn't quite strong enough. You'll ruin the whole batch, extracting all the substances you wanted to leave behind in the grounds. If you must, pour weak coffee through freshly ground coffee.

Burner Remedies: Thermal Carafes

Nothing is more destructive to good coffee than the burners on coffee machines. A burner is aptly named. It ruins brewed coffee as soon as it starts dripping into the carafe, overheating it and throwing the flavor completely out of balance. Burners are today's national disgrace—the chief reason you don't like most coffee you are served. Coffee should be held at about 185 degrees F and not on a burner, which vaporizes many desirable aromatics, oxidizes oils and leaves coffee sour or bitter.

The solution is to transfer coffee to an insulated carafe as soon as it is brewed. *If you want to keep brewed coffee hot, the only way without ruining it is to put it into a thermal carafe.* Be sure to preheat the carafe with hot water or the cold glass lining will instantly cool your fresh, hot coffee.

Some insulated carafes look clumsy, and some look stylish and streamlined. Several Japanese makers have designed handsome brushed-aluminum carafes that hold only about three large cups of coffee, a convenient size. When using any insulated carafe, the goal is to have as airtight a seal as possible: the less air at the top of the inner chamber, the longer the liquid will stay hot. You should buy a carafe that holds no more than the amount of coffee you usually brew at one time.

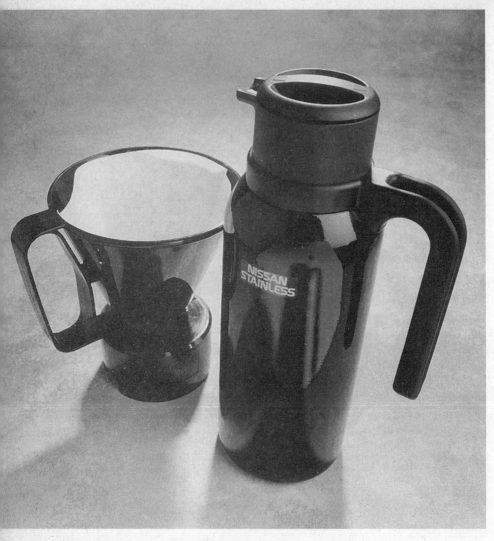

Manual drip filter holder and thermal carafe

The best innovation in electric drip brewers is the substitution of thermal for glass carafes, abolishing the evil burner. This is the only kind of electric brewer a coffee lover can recommend with a clear conscience, although it's unfortunately difficult to find one with a high-wattage rating. (The Technivorm is one.)

A thermal carafe won't give brewed coffee everlasting life, even if many coffee bars think that "air pots" (big insulated carafes into which commercial brewers drip coffee) can sit on a counter all day long. Just because coffee is hot doesn't mean it's good, as the expert Kevin Knox points out. A rule for tasting only what's good is to toss out any coffee more than forty minutes old.

Although it's best not to reheat cold coffee, you can at least heat it up without destroying the coffee. The microwave oven has come to the rescue. Its very inefficiency in boiling liquid is an advantage for coffee and milk, both of which taste terrible boiled. If you're reheating in a cardboard or Styrofoam cup, leave it uncovered: the cover often warps, since it wasn't designed to go into a microwave oven. Still, there's no substitute for freshly brewed coffee.

When shopping for an electric brewer, then, look for a machine with a wattage of over 1,000 and a thermal carafe instead of a glass one. For ordinary electric drip brewers, pretend that the brew-interrupt feature is broken and that if you interrupt the cycle, coffee will overflow everywhere. Pretend, too, that the burner doesn't work and that the only thing to do is to transfer brewed coffee immediately to a thermal carafe. It won't keep forever. Consider forty minutes to be the maximum holding time.

Defiantly Simple:
The Manual Filter Method

What, really, are you paying for when you buy an electric drip machine? The answer, I think, is that you're paying to walk away. But it takes very little additional time or trouble to brew with a defiantly low-tech arrangement: a plastic filter holder that fits snugly over a thermal carafe. Kits whose carafes hold about a quart of liquid are readily available at coffee stores for about $25, whereas a high-end electric brewer runs $80 or even over $150. These simple devices may not be quite as stylish as electric machines, but they're sturdy and, at least in black, pretty good-looking.

The manual filter method, to give it a dignified name, neatly avoids all the traps of the electric brewer. You can be sure the water temperature is right by waiting a few seconds after you remove the whistling kettle from the stove. You can stick to the Brewing Proportions (page 93), using nothing more specialized than measuring cups. You can pour the water through the ground coffee in a way that will guarantee even saturation, so that the water will take the best from the grounds and you can avoid the problem of overflow. You can be sure that the brewed coffee won't be destroyed by sitting on a burner.

Filter holders come in many sizes and will fit over many cups and mugs. Whatever container the coffee is dripping into should be rinsed first in very hot or boiling water. The headroom rule still applies when you're measuring ground coffee into the filter: if the grounds come up pretty high in the filter, simply pour in the water in stages. A good tip is to buy paper filters one size larger than recommended, so that you won't have to worry that water will overflow and run down the sides of the filter holder.

Pouring water in by stages is always a good idea. Premoistening creates an evenly resistant bed for the remaining water, which will travel through the

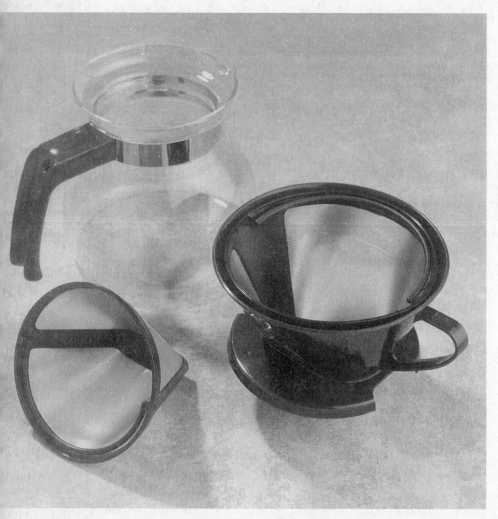

Melitta brewer, gold filters and glass carafe

grounds at a consistent rate instead of zipping through the channels that can form if all the water is poured on at once. If you're using ½ cup of ground coffee, moisten the grounds first with ½ cup of hot water, trying to wet them evenly, and wait 30 seconds before pouring in the rest of the liquid (in this case, 2½ cups) all at once, assuming the filter is big enough. If the coffee was roasted recently, you'll see the lovely puffing dome that professional cuppers see dozens of times a day.

You can tell that the brewing has been uneven if, after the water passes through the grounds, you see little holes at the top, like the holes in rice after it steams or in sand after the tide rolls out. You should instead see a flat bed. An extra precaution is to stir together the grounds and water after you add all the water to the filter, which you should then cover while the water finishes seeping through. Swirl the liquid to amalgamate the brew, and serve yourself and anyone at hand.

In the 1960s, the German company Melitta began marketing a coffee maker in the United States with a wedge-shaped filter holder and filters that open like a pocket, so the water passes through only one layer of paper. The company, which takes its name from Melitta Bentz, a woman who devised a paper filter drip machine in 1908, first sold the pocket-wedge filters in the 1930s in Germany; before then, filters were usually hand-folded. Today, the wedge shape dominates the market, and it is available in the widest range of sizes. You can buy paper or, better, metal filters in one- and two-cup sizes: the wedge is a good size for small quantities, because the small volume of grounds will form the deepest and most resistant bed for the hot water. (A flat basket is more efficient for large quantities.)

Lab Appeal: The Chemex

Although my ideal brewing equipment is a filter holder over a thermal carafe, other manual drip methods are still in use, and they're perfectly legitimate. Paper filters first reached the wide attention of American coffee lovers in the mid-1930s, when a German-born scientist and inventor named Peter Schlumbohm introduced the Chemex, a handblown glass coffee maker with an hourglass shape. The Chemex looks like it came straight from a laboratory, which it more or less did, and has a stark, International Style cachet. This is a style, like that of the German Bauhaus, in which everything is severely functional

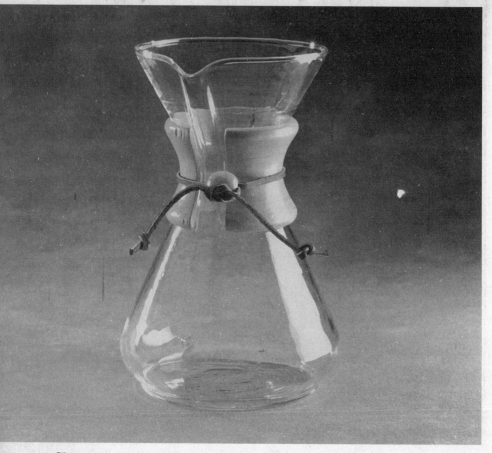

Chemex

and usually made of glass, steel or concrete; it was radical between the wars, and by the 1950s was synonymous with modern design. The Chemex is still available in most specialty-coffee stores, although it doesn't offer any advantages over other manual filters except looks.

Certainly the original Chemex is handsome. A cheaper model, made of machine-blown rather than handblown glass and with a useful glass handle at the waist replacing the old wooden cuffs bound with a leather drawstring, is less striking. But the Chemex is a pain to clean. You need to buy S-shaped bottle brushes to wash out the bottom half. Worse, because the filter paper is sold in sheets (either circles or squares) that are folded into quarters and set into the cone-shaped upper half, part of the coffee goes through three layers of paper.

This is coffee that's too pure. You can buy cone-shaped gold-washed metal filters, but I don't see the point of buying a Chemex unless you're an architect or you like the lab look. There's no advantage in the fact that the heat-tempered glass can sit over a low flame: a flame is just what you shouldn't subject brewed coffee to.

Theatrical Brewing: The Neapolitan Flip

If I know I won't want more than two generous cups of coffee, I often use a sentimental favorite—a metal flip-drip pot that in France is called the *café filtre* and in Italy the *napoletana,* or Neapolitan machine (many American shops call it a *macchinetta*). It has two cylindrical pots, one atop the other,

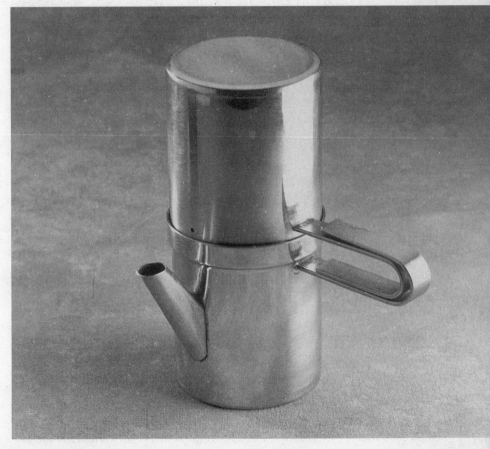

Neapolitan flip

one with a spout. Between them neatly fits a separate compartment for ground coffee, with metal screens at the top and bottom.

The method is a bit theatrical. You fill the lower, spoutless chamber with water and set it to boil. When the water has boiled, turn off the heat, wait a few seconds for it to cool a bit, put in the insert containing the coffee grounds, and latch on the top half, whose spout will be upside down. (Italians latch the machine before putting it on the stove. I prefer to keep an eye on the water.) Then flip the whole thing over and take it off the heat or set it on a heat diffuser while the coffee drips. (No water leaks out during the dramatic flip —the latch is secure.) After three minutes or so, the water has dripped through. As with all filtered coffee, the finished brew should be stirred before it is served, because the coffee that drips through first is strongest.

The napoletana is very like good old American drip pots, which are still sold in hardware stores. For many people, the clunky design, with its squat stacked compartments for hot water, ground coffee and brewed coffee, brings back childhood. Unfortunately, most drip pots are made of aluminum, which interacts with the acid in coffee. This is a problem with the napoletana, too, but you can find stainless steel pots (see Sources, page 254).

I prefer the napoletana to the American drip, not just because I like flipping the pot but also because I like the relatively high ratio of ground coffee (3 scoops) to water (1½ cups). The incised cup markings on the filter basket and water chamber of an old-fashioned drip pot are usually misleading, and you should measure out both the coffee and water. The napoletana requires a medium-coarse grind; the holes in the screens of American pots are generally smaller, so you can use a medium-fine grind. Remember, just because these pots are heat-resistant doesn't mean you should keep them on the heat.

Italians so closely identify with the napoletana that they wish they could take credit for it, even though they didn't really invent it (the French did). A book on the history of the pot published by Alessi, the tableware designer that once made the handsomest one (it was discontinued), is full of illustrations of fanciful napoletanas that look like robots, or wear masks, or are gotten up like top-hatted dancers with canes. The book says that every resident of Naples knows you can't make decent coffee in a new napoletana. It's wrong. A residue of coffee oils is unpleasant in any kind of pot and is a particular danger with a metal one—the oil becomes rancid. Metal pots, like everything else used to brew coffee, should be regularly scrubbed in hot water.

Rich Results: The Plunger Pot

Infusion has an appealing directness. It's absolutely plain, like steeping tea leaves in water. This is, after all, how cuppers, the world's most discerning coffee connoisseurs, evaluate coffee. Chief among the merits of steeped coffee is thicker body than even my cherished napoletana, with its wide holes in a metal screen, can offer.

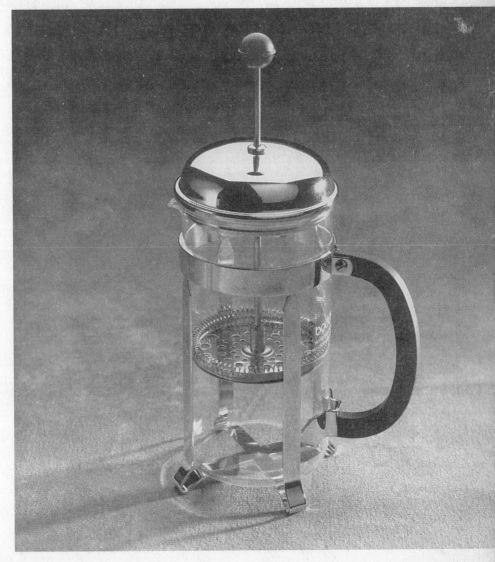

Bodum plunger pot

Infusion survives today in three forms. The most primitive—open-pot coffee, also called cowboy, campfire or hobo coffee—is made by strewing ground coffee over water that has come to a boil and leaving it to steep for five minutes or so. It can be strained through cloth or nylon mesh or even a sock, part of campfire legend. Or you can add cold water in the hope that the grounds will settle; they won't completely. Many people, especially the ones who scorn fancy appliances, swear by open-pot coffee. I find the straining more trouble than it's worth.

The easiest way to steep coffee is in a plunger pot. It produces a strong brew with a fair amount of sediment, depending on the fineness of the wire-strainer mesh and of the grind; these pots require a coarse grind. One reason the plunger pot is becoming ever more popular is that it is at its best with beans of a fairly dark roast, the kind now popular. As with espresso, plunger-pot coffee highlights acidity to a degree that can be distracting with a medium-light roast.

The Danish company Bodum makes several lines of plunger pots in appealing designs. All have similar glass cylinders and screens of plastic, nylon or metal, depending on the price. Aficionados claim that the machines are not nearly as well made as when Melior produced them in France (Bodum bought the company); the screens aren't as finely tooled, they complain, and leave room at the sides of the carafe. Alessi makes the best-looking version, a Michael Graves design with a shiny stainless-steel carafe holder in open squares like something from 1920s Vienna. At about $140 for the eight-cup pot, it is expensive but both attractive and solid (see Sources, page 253).

The pots can be tricky to use. The suspended grounds have so much surface tension that the effort of getting the plunger to the bottom can lift your feet off the floor, and the problem is worse if the coffee was ground too fine. If you push down the plunger at an angle—the spindle is thin, and it's hard to push exactly straight—you can break the carafe. Fishing out the grounds from the bottom when you go to clean the pot is annoying. Worst, by the time the coffee has finished steeping, it has cooled, a problem remedied only partly by the quilted plunger-pot cozies that specialty-coffee shops sell or by wrapping a terry-cloth towel around the pot, a trick I learned from Martha Stewart.

Still, a plunger pot offers the richest coffee this side of espresso, and for around $15, it's certainly worth trying one out. Rinse the carafe in hot water before adding the coffee; the best results come from a larger quantity than usual of coarse-ground coffee (see Brewing Proportions, page 93). Let the slightly cooled boiling water steep with the grounds for four to six minutes. I prefer a full six minutes; others stop at five. Do something else while waiting: a watched pot never steeps. Then slowly and carefully push the screen to the bottom of the pot. If you mean to hold the coffee for more than ten minutes or so, transfer it to a thermal carafe to keep it warm. A few manufacturers even offer metal plunger pots with thermal walls.

The third form in which infusion survives is coffee made with cold water. This method becomes fashionable every few years and then retreats into deserved obscurity. People are drawn to it because the coffee is low in acid and because it produces an extract that works as a kind of homemade instant coffee. A pound of ground coffee steeps in a quart of cold water for ten to twenty-four hours and is then filtered through a funnel-like device. The resulting extract, which is stirred into hot water, is mild and characterless, because cold water does not extract the lighter aromatics or acids in coffee —or the oils, or much of anything. But it's inoffensive mixed with milk as a kind of soft drink, and can be of help to people who suffer upset stomachs when they drink coffee. The funnel kits cost about $30, so you can try the method when, for instance, you know you'll want to make lots of iced coffee for a picnic. Otherwise, it's a novelty you probably won't try again.

Museum Piece: The Percolator

Any kind of metal filter—gold, stainless steel or aluminum—is necessary for true percolation, which is the filtering of liquid through a metal or even a ceramic screen. I believe strongly in metal filters. Why, then, do I consider electric or stovetop percolators to be fit only for museums of American household life? Because they commit an unpardonable crime: they boil coffee.

Until the late eighteenth century, European coffee meant boiled coffee. Boiling persisted as the chief mode of brewing in both Europe and the United States easily until the 1930s, in the face of many superior methods. Writing in the United States in the 1920s, William H. Ukers, the author of *All About Coffee,* an encyclopedia that is still a standard reference work, called boiled coffee a "crying evil."

He was right, of course. Boiling coffee is the fastest way to drive off delicate aromatics, and it only heightens the bitter and sour components. Small wonder that the English, in their legendary eighteenth-century coffeehouses, where the essay and modern prose style were honed, laced their boiled coffee with sugar, egg yolk and all manner of strong-flavored ingredients, including mustard. The Dutch, according to the author Ian Bersten, would, in the mid-nineteenth century, roast coffee beans with cocoa beans, lemon pips, cinnamon or bread—and if the beans looked in some way damaged, they substituted an onion for the bread and added cloves and peppercorns.

Americans unfortunately adopted the pumping percolator, which was the only really harmful innovation coming out of an extraordinarily inventive period in early nineteenth-century France, when the forerunners of the drip and filter machines we use today were patented at a feverish rate. The pumping percolator forces boiling water up through a tube and sprays it over the grounds. This would be fine, if the process stopped there. But the weak brew from the first pass is repeatedly boiled to create enough steam pressure to force it back up the tube, and liquid is sprayed over the grounds again and again until it darkens. Meanwhile, most of the aromatics are burned off and the rest are oxidized, and the coffee is horribly overextracted.

It's true that few things are as cheering or welcoming as the "perking of the coffee right nearby," as Frank Loesser's lyric has it in the jaunty 1941 song "I Hear Music." You shouldn't storm out of a house where perked coffee is served. Better to be served coffee perked from a just-opened can of ground supermarket coffee, poured as soon as it's finished, than to drink coffee brewed in an electric drip machine from "gourmet" beans that have been sitting for weeks in a Lucite bin, then poured after two hours of sitting on a burner. At the house of a friend who swears by perked coffee, I recently gave it a fair shake. I can report that the percolator just isn't a good choice for making coffee—like boiled coffee, perked coffee is out of balance and acrid.

Middle Eastern Method: Boiling Coffee

Nordic countries still boil coffee, as people still do in Lake Wobegon country, with its Scandinavian heritage. The method is not only harmful to decent coffee but cumbersome besides. It starts out simpler than the percolator: all you do is boil coffee grounds in water. Things get difficult at the end. Separating out the grounds requires messy and tedious steps like casting egg shells or raw egg whites over the surface, which will attract the grounds and form a scum you can skim off.

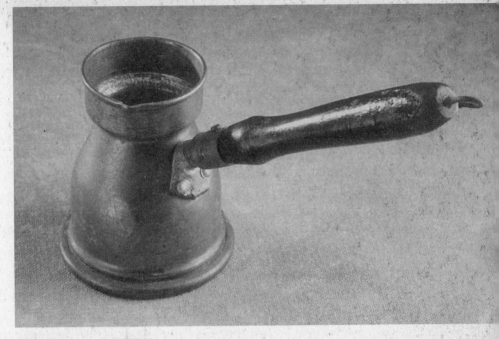

Turkish cezve (briki)

One instance of boiling coffee actually produces something that tastes good, or at any rate something I like to drink: Turkish, or Greek, coffee. Be careful what you call it, because patriots of either country will take offense if you use the wrong name. Kenneth Davids, in *Coffee,* proposes a diplomatic name, "Middle Eastern coffee." It is said to have originated in the coffeehouses of Cairo in the fifteenth century. Whatever the name, the method is similar throughout the Mideast, although different countries have their own variations. The coffee is boiled several times in a long-handled brass or copper pot, tinned on the interior, which slopes inward at the top. Today the pot is called a *cezve* (pronounced "jezwe") in Turkey; in American shops it usually goes by its original name, *ibrik,* which survives as the Greek *briki.* The froth—the sign of an expert maker—is distributed equally among the guests.

Middle Eastern coffee requires the finest grind of any kind of coffee, because the grounds are never strained out. It's as fine as cake flour, and home grinders simply can't produce it. If you can't find a briki or cezve at a specialty shop, buy an identically shaped pot, usually enameled and sold for heating butter, which is easy to find. You can buy specially ground coffee at

Greek, Arab or Turkish food or spice shops, or ask your local bean shop to grind a light-roast coffee at the very finest setting. Rinse a demitasse cup or two in hot water; you won't get more than two cups out of the standard cezve. If you have a proper Turkish coffee cup—it resembles a small eggcup in a metal stand—so much the better. Use about 2 teaspoons of the powdery ground beans to ½ cup of water. Stir in as much sugar as you like (the usual dose in the Middle East is equal parts sugar and ground coffee) and put the coffee over a medium flame. Bring the liquid coffee to a frothing simmer. Just as it puffs and is about to boil over, remove it from the stove and pour a bit of foam into the cup or cups.

Everyone prizes the foam, but don't get your hopes up: not everyone achieves it. Getting the foam right, in fact, is said to be the test of a prospective daughter-in-law on her first visit to her beau's mother. To finish the process, bring the coffee back to the simmer once more—or repeat twice more, to duplicate Greek practice—and pour out the rest.

People think of Middle Eastern coffee as dreadfully strong and muddy. But the mud settles to the bottom of the cup pretty fast, and the remaining liquid is surprisingly sweet and mild, probably because fairly insipid beans are commonly used and they are roasted very light. Also, the actual boiling is minimal—the adage, commonly and correctly used in Turkey, is that boiled coffee is spoiled coffee. So, for that matter, is the entire contact time of coffee and water. The point is to produce the froth. Whether you do or not, you'll find that the coffee is altogether more pleasant than you might have imagined.

Alchemical Purity: The Vacuum Pot

When you've tried the rest and you want to try the best—even if you might not try it very often—you can have fun with the most dramatic way to make filtered coffee. The peculiar-looking vacuum pot was invented in Germany in the mid-nineteenth century, and in several versions it looked even more peculiar than it does today. The model most commonly available has two glass globes, one set into the other with a filter between the two, suspended over a spirit lamp or other heat source.

These machines became fashionable in America around the First World War and fell out of favor in the 1950s. For a time, they were standard even in luncheonettes, where they were known as Silex machines, after the commonest U.S. manufacturer. Another maker gave its name to the method—Cona, an English company that still produces the best and handsomest model. The Cona machine is expensive, from about $150 to $250, depending on size, and hard to find (see Sources, page 253). Bodum, the Scandinavian manufacturer, has been a strong advocate of the vacuum pot since the mid-1950s, when Peter Bodum introduced the pot into Denmark. The company still makes a stovetop model for about $40 and one with a spirit lamp for about $20 more. Its great innovation has been to design a sleek, transparent plastic vacuum coffee maker that is completely electric, down to a programmable timer and dishwasher-safe carafes to make it compete with electric drip machines. The 12-cup model of the Santos, for about $100 (first sold by Starbucks in the United States as the Utopia), takes up more counter room than other electric drip machines, but the handsome new 6-cup Santos (about $60), with two off-set chambers, is just the right size and offers all the requisite ease of operation to show anyone why I call vacuum pots the key to enjoying the full flavor spectrum of a fine bean.

For the spectacular, if cumbersome, pre-electric method, you first set water to boil in a kettle (don't follow instructions to boil over a spirit lamp, which will take hours). Latch into the base of the upper globe the filter provided—either glass, plastic or metal, depending on the manufacturer. Pour whatever quantity the manufacturer recommends of finely ground coffee into the globe (the top is open); sizes vary by model. The ground coffee sits dry and loose around the filter.

Now the alchemy can begin. Set the lower globe on the stand and fill it with hot water. Fit the upper globe, which has a tube protruding from the filter, snugly into the lower globe, creating an airtight seal, and set the assembled machine over a low flame. Steam pressure forces the water up through the tube into the upper globe, where you stir the ground coffee with the water. It looks like sludge. Wait two minutes or so for the coffee to steep, then extinguish the flame. As the air in the lower globe cools and contracts, a vacuum forms, sucking the slurry through the filter and back into the bottom globe with a gurgling whoosh that will surprise and delight guests. Remove the upper globe and ceremoniously pour the coffee.

The whole rigmarole is best performed in the parlor after dinner rather than in the kitchen before you've had your morning coffee, and it looks like a

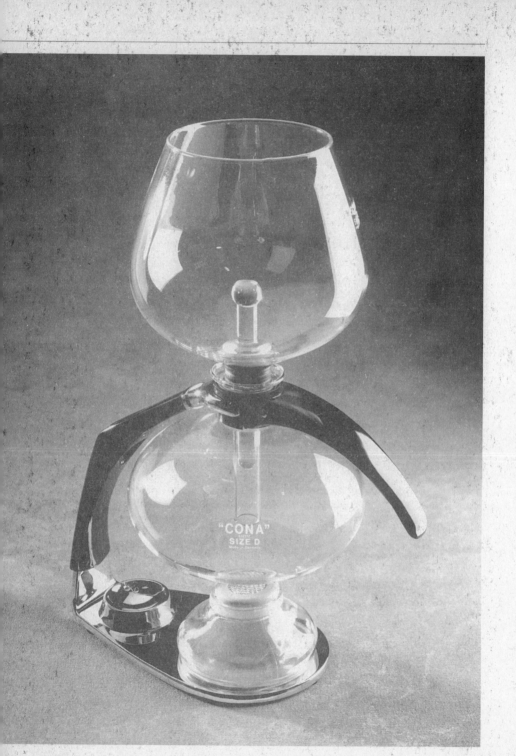

Cona glass vacuum PotMoka stovetop brewer

road-show magician's act. But it's a matchless way to sample a fine coffee with complex acidity—no other brewing method better showcases high flavor notes. The several steps mean that you will use a vacuum pot very seldom. But this is coffee at its purest and most lyrical. And anyone who watches you make it will think you know everything there is to know about brewing.

BREWING PROPORTIONS

These are the ratios of ground coffee to water that I find make the best brewed coffee. They apply to any filtering method, using paper or gold filters. (For vacuum pots, follow the manufacturer's suggestions.)

I proceed by scoops of coffee (be sure your scoop holds a full 2 tablespoons; many scoops today hold just one), because it's the most important measurement in an electric drip machine, the method most people use. The chart ends with the maximum amount of ground coffee most machines can handle. Ground coffee retains a good deal of water, so the yield is surprisingly lower than the water you start with.

Because the cup lines on the carafes of electric drip machines vary, my advice is to use standard kitchen measuring cups to fill the carafe or reservoir, depending on your habit, and to note for the future the level that the water reaches.

GROUND COFFEE	WATER	BREWED COFFEE
¼ cup (2 scoops)	1 cup (8 oz.)	¾ cup (6 oz.)
¼ cup + 2 tablespoons (3 scoops)	2 cups (16 oz.)	1½ cups (12 oz.)
½ cup (4 scoops)	3 cups (24 oz.)	2¼ cups (18 oz.)
½ cup + 2 tablespoons (5 scoops)	3½ cups (28 oz.)	2¾ cups (22 oz.)
¾ cup (6 scoops)	4 cups (32 oz.)	3 cups (24 oz.)
¾ cup + 2 tablespoons (7 scoops)	4½ cups (36 oz.)	3½ cups (28 oz.)
1 cup (8 scoops)	5½ cups (44 oz.)	4½ cups (36 oz.)
1 cup + 2 tablespoons (9 scoops)	6¼ cups (50 oz.)	4¾ cups (38 oz.)

BREWING AT A GLANCE

Electric Drip

ADVANTAGES: Produces acceptable drip coffee almost by itself. Best way short of big urns to make coffee for a crowd.

DISADVANTAGES: Filter basket can overflow even if the correct amount of ground coffee is used, especially if it's freshly roasted and ground. Most machines are designed to brew with water that isn't hot enough and take too long to brew. Burners keep coffee hot but ruin it.

LOOK FOR: Thermal carafes instead of glass pots. Wattage ratings of at least 850 and preferably 1,000 watts. Gold-washed metal filters that fit into the basket as a substitute for paper filters.

BUY: A thermal carafe and metal filter if the machine doesn't come with them. Also, packets of cleaning powder to be run through the machine's brew cycle once a month.

GRIND: Medium to medium-coarse.

BREW TIPS: Stir the moistened grounds in the filter basket if the machine allows access to the basket. Don't steal a cup before the whole pot is brewed. Swirl the pot to stir the coffee before pouring the first cup. Keep the coffee warm in a thermal carafe, never on a burner.

Manual Drip

ADVANTAGES: Really easy. Portable. Offers complete control over water temperature and coffee-to-water ratio.

DISADVANTAGES: Takes slightly longer than electric drip, because you boil water separately and stand over the filter to pour it through.

LOOK FOR: A large filter holder that fits into a thermal carafe.

BUY: A metal filter insert to fit the filter holder. Oversized paper filters, if you prefer paper.

GRIND: Medium for paper filters. Medium-fine for metal filters.

BREW TIPS: Rinse the thermal carafe or the cup you will brew into with hot water first. Let boiling water rest for fifteen to twenty seconds before pouring it over ground coffee. Moisten grounds thoroughly with a portion of the hot water, waiting thirty seconds for it to soak in before adding the rest of the water. Add the rest all at once, or as much at a time as will fit into the filter without overflowing. Cover the filter holder to prevent heat loss. Swirl the final brew before serving.

Flip-Drip and American Metal Drip

ADVANTAGES: Richer body of coffee made with metal rather than paper filter. Italian flip-drip pots take a higher than usual amount of ground coffee to water, producing a strong but not harsh cup. Flipping the pot is fun.

DISADVANTAGES: Coffee must be transferred to a thermal carafe if you don't plan to drink it right away. Coffee measurements incised into American drip pots are usually wrong. Some people dislike any sediment at the bottom of their cup; all metal filters leave a little.

LOOK FOR: Stainless steel and not aluminum, which interacts with coffee acids to produce off flavors. Heatproof handles on flip-drip pots.

GRIND: Medium-coarse for flip-drip; medium-fine for American drip.

BREW TIPS: Don't overfill the flip-drip chamber with grounds. Let boiling water rest for fifteen to twenty seconds before brewing. Swirl the final brew before serving.

Plunger Pot

ADVANTAGES: Richest body this side of espresso, resulting from the high ratio of coffee to water, the steeping time and the slight application of pressure.

DISADVANTAGES: Sediment at the bottom of the cup. Coffee cools as it steeps and quickly thereafter. A chore to clean if you don't have a dishwasher.

LOOK FOR: A metal filter screen, not nylon mesh. A tight fit of filter screen into glass container. A wide knob for pushing down the screen, which will ensure even pressure and reduce the risk of breaking the carafe.

GRIND: Coarse.

BREW TIPS: Rinse the glass container with hot water first. Wrap a terry-cloth towel around the pot during steeping.

Middle Eastern Coffee

ADVANTAGES: Thick body, surprisingly mild flavor. Entertaining brewing process.

DISADVANTAGES: A great deal of sediment at the bottom of the cup. Brief boiling, which robs delicate beans of much of their flavor.

BUY: A slope-sided, long-handled open pot, often called an ibrik, or any pot the same shape, such as the enameled ones sold for warming butter and milk. Light-roasted beans from Central America or Africa.

GRIND: Extremely fine.

BREW TIPS: Bring just to a simmering boil two or three times, depending on whether you want to emulate Turkish or Greek practice (two for Turkish, three for Greek), and pour immediately into small cups.

Vacuum Pot

ADVANTAGES: The compact disc of coffees. Utterly pure, delivering the very best of what a fine coffee has to give.

DISADVANTAGES: Finicky and time-consuming.

LOOK FOR: A pot that can go over a stove or, to save time but not counter space, an electric model. Classic models have cloth filters, which produce a clearer brew than plastic ones.

GRIND: Medium-fine.

BREW TIPS: Boil water separately to avoid spending all day. Stir the mixture of coffee grounds and water in the upper globe before removing from the heat source, at which point the vacuum is created. Serve immediately in order to taste the coffee at its best; the remarkably clear coffee will also keep very well in a thermal carafe.

6 | Espresso

I T DOESN'T MATTER HOW SMALL a town in Italy is. Even if it looks as though a delivery truck comes through only once a month, you'll find an espresso bar. There will be a hodgepodge of tables where people can play cards or hold court, and maybe a miniature soccer game in the corner. In short, the bar defines the center of town.

Because Italians so love their coffee, and because we so love things Italian, we assume that they must love particularly good coffee. This isn't necessarily so. Italians love coffee made a certain way—a way that gets the very most out of beans, whatever their quality. The difference is the brewing method: forcing hot but not boiling water *at high pressure* through finely ground beans, fast.

Nothing matches the thickness of true espresso. The pressure forces the water to emulsify with the oils and proteins naturally present in coffee, just as, with mayonnaise, oil emulsifies with egg yolks, lemon juice and air to produce a thick, creamy sauce. The result is a syrupy liquid whose flavor rolls onto the tongue like a tide slowly coming in, completely overtaking the palate and lingering for twenty minutes or so.

Espresso came to its greatest glory in Italy, and during a century's worth of invention, tinkerers competed to serve the country's expanding thirst not just for espresso but for morning cappuccino, made with espresso and milk that has been foamed to a cashmere softness by the injection of steam.

The requirements for the bittersweet miracle of espresso are many. Certainly, blend, roast, quality and freshness of beans are crucial. But they won't translate into the blast that makes Italians regularly stop everything for sixty seconds to down "six drops of energy," as an Italian friend once aptly summarized a shot of espresso, unless the machine is in perfect running order and in expert hands.

If beans are freshly roasted or out of the can without having been exposed to light and air for many days, and the ground beans are properly fine but not floury, and the water is the right temperature (about twenty degrees below boiling), and every part of the machine is preheated and the china cup preheated, too, and if the operator has a sense of improvisation born of long experience, then the six drops will be blessed with a layer of tan foam called crema.

Crema, which looks like fine sea spray, is the Holy Grail of espresso, the beautifully tangible sign that everything has gone right. It's hard to achieve with anything less than a professional espresso machine—a glorious piece of equipment as temperamental as a sports car, born of the Italian love of technology that turns a doodle into a diagram.

The Italian *barista,* the master of the espresso machine, usually has a deeper attachment to the streamlined box behind the bar than to any other machine in his life (*barista* means "barman," and most baristas are men). Nothing about it can be taken for granted, not ever. Meticulous daily cleaning and tiny adjustments in the espresso machine and, especially, the grinder are what keep crema on top of the cup.

"Made to Order" at the Bar

Espresso first became popular around the turn of the century, and the only places that served it were bars. The very idea of custom-made coffee was unusual: for decades the norm had been big boiled urns full of weakish brew. Most historians explain the meaning of "espresso" with regard to coffee as "made to order"; the word also means "fast," as in mail delivery. Huge, fur-nacelike contraptions, often sprouting eagles and other elaborate sculptural ornaments, dominated coffeehouses like altars. The machines had to be huge: only big boilers could build up enough steam pressure to force hot water repeatedly through ground coffee to turn out espresso after espresso.

The true potential of espresso was realized only in 1948, when Giovanni Achille Gaggia, a Milanese barman born in 1895, wrought a revolution. His machine had a spring-powered piston mounted right over the filter holder, the detachable part that holds the ground coffee. The piston pushed hot water through the coffee at over 100 pounds per square inch. This meant a sweeter and much more powerful cup of coffee. Ian Bersten, in his pathbreaking his-tory of coffee drinking and coffee machines, *Coffee Floats, Tea Sinks,* calls Gaggia's spring-powered piston machine "perhaps the single biggest develop-ment of all time in coffee brewing."

A mechanical source of pressure also meant that water could be forced through the coffee at any temperature, rather than at or close to the boil, as in steam machines. Specialists had long known that it is best not to let boiling water near ground coffee beans: it scalds them and extracts bitter substances. Water at fifteen or twenty degrees below the boil provides the best extraction.

The twin improvements of greatly increased pressure and a suitable water temperature had enormous consequences—and all of them could be read at the top of the cup. Gaggia noticed that his machine produced a mousselike layer of beige foam. Many coffee-shop owners to whom he excitedly demonstrated this marvelous, odd substance scorned it as strange scum. But Gaggia knew he had found something new and wonderful.

Gaggia died in 1961, the year of the next and perhaps last epochal machine—the Faema E61, named for a 1961 eclipse. The Faema E61, all chrome and pressure gauges and rhomboid biomorphic shapes, was made by Ernesto Valente, a rival of Gaggia's. It relied on an electric pump rather than a spring-loaded piston. The pump forces cool, fresh tap water through a spiral copper pipe mounted inside a boiler full of hot water. Still pushed by the pump, the newly heated water in the pipe travels straight through the ground coffee and into the espresso cup.

The boiler of the Faema and all modern espresso machines is used to heat fresh water for espresso and to produce steam for milk. Today, the simplest home espresso machines still use steam pressure to force hot water through the ground coffee, as in the early days of bar espresso; better home machines use pistons or pumps to do the forcing. But what touches the ground coffee is hot water—not steam. Steam would disastrously scald ground coffee, whereas it does wondrous things to milk.

All the home espresso machines worth investing in are outgrowths of the Gaggia and Faema landmarks. Even if home espresso machines have little of the visual panache of barroom speedsters, they can reward you with a rich, satisfying, utterly delicious few sips of coffee. They also offer the way to make satiny foamed milk—milk that tastes like nothing you've had before in your kitchen. Though cheaper than their bar forerunners, which cost thousands of dollars, these home versions, known broadly as "pump machines," are still expensive—$200 and up, with the most solid models priced at $350 to $400.

Low-Tech Solutions: The Moka

Before you take out a loan, consider the coffee-making method that has been popular in Italy for more than half a century—one that will require a layout of less than $30.

Italians themselves almost never bother trying to duplicate their several-times-a-day bar experience at home. What they use to make coffee is an easy, inexpensive, time-tested stovetop brewer called the *moka*, popularized in the thirties by its first large-scale manufacturer, Bialetti. The choice of "Moka" as a brand name was arbitrary, and had nothing to do with chocolate or a port on the Arabian Peninsula from which beans were shipped. It resulted in yet another meaning of the word "mocha," this one coffee brewed in such a pot. In steam machines, as the moka and all its cousins, some of them electric-powered, are generically called, water boils in a closed chamber with enough headroom to allow a head of steam to collect. The pressure from the steam forces the hot water out of the chamber and through the ground coffee. (The steam is just for the pressure; as with all forms of espresso, hot water and not steam comes into contact with the coffee.)

What comes out is drip coffee with a push. The force of gravity equals one "bar," the measurement of pressure. Drip coffee brews at a little over one bar (it drips). The ideal pressure for espresso is nine bars. A steam machine like the moka brews at between one and a half and three bars, enough to add some texture and to produce some of the emulsion that gives true espresso its thickness and flavor. Some shops say that steam machines produce double-strength coffee, which isn't far off the mark. Italians call what they make at home *caffè*. They know that it isn't true espresso, and that's okay. Even if coffee from a moka is almost never crowned by crema, it works well enough for milk drinks.

I'm almost irrationally attached to the moka, for its associations with every Italian household I've ever visited and also because it's so simple and reliable. The design hasn't changed since its introduction in 1933: faceted

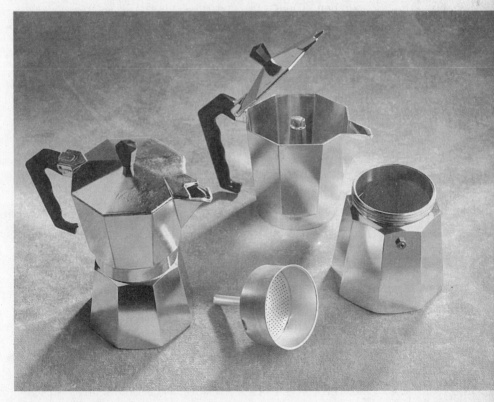

Moka stovetop brewer

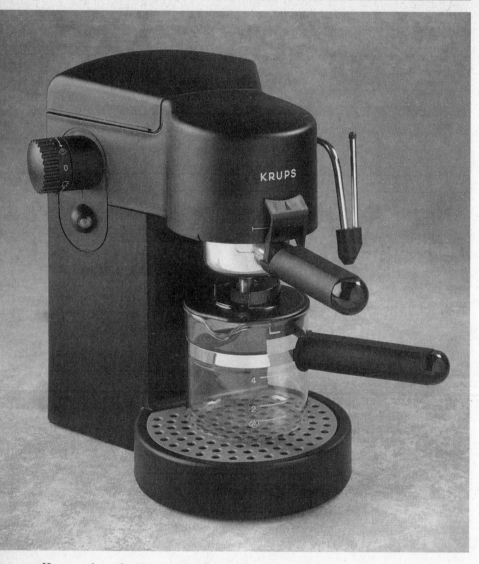

Krups electric steam machine

metal upper and lower chambers with a cinched waist where the coffee filter goes. Brewers of this shape are unfortunately made of aluminum, which is always dangerous around coffee, because it interacts with the acids in coffee and produces off flavors. Stainless-steel versions are fairly easy to find (see Sources, page 255). They come in less evocative shapes and fewer sizes—the commonest is for three to four cups of espresso, whereas in the classic you find twelve-cup models—but they don't darken and pit, as aluminum brewers do. In Italian-American shops, you occasionally find mokas of the classic cinched-waist design with ceramic upper chambers, which confer a gentler heat to the coffee; the only such pots I've seen are covered with kitschy blue flowers.

The method brings compromises, starting with the extraction of bitter substances from coffee by near-boiling water. Also, with a very few exceptions, you can't brew one cup at a time. This can be an advantage when serving a small crowd, because you get all the brewing out of the way at once. Mokas are not for those who want perfect espresso, but they are boons to those who care about convenience and thrift. They are easy to clean, and they take up little space; their only maintenance is an occasional replacement gasket, which is available at most stores that sell the pots. (See Using a Moka, page 117.)

Electric steam machines work just like the moka but are priced between $80 and $100. The extra money is for an electric heat source and for styling to make it look professional. Electric steam machines also come equipped with a milk-steaming nozzle, but it's generally useless: once the steam pressure in the small boiler pushes hot water through the ground coffee, there's rarely enough pressure left to foam the milk properly.

Even if I dismiss electric steam machines, most stores and most shoppers do not. The machines look just like pump machines except smaller. Don't be fooled by the professional-looking apparatus and the sleek design. These offer few advantages over a stovetop moka. A better investment is an electric milk steamer to accompany a moka, which for about $70 will enable you to make perfectly acceptable cappuccino and *caffelatte*, the Italian family drink that appears on American espresso-bar menus as "caffè latte."

Designed to Impress: The Pavoni

Of the high-priced machines capable of giving you a cup of real espresso, the home piston machine made by the Italian firm Pavoni is the most labor-intensive. It is a chromed or brass-plated wonder, bristling with domestic-sized versions of the boilers, rubber-coated handles, tubes and levers found on espresso-bar machines. So splendid is it and so clearly does it announce that its owner truly cares about espresso that some espresso-machine shoppers decide nothing else will do. This decision will bring much grief, a considerably

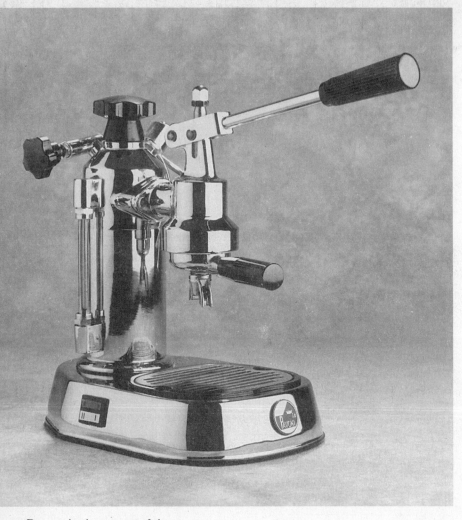

Pavoni piston machine

lightened bank account (the Pavoni costs at least $400) and an eventual search for a spot on a high shelf.

You're paying for a functioning antique. The Pavoni is a throwback to the pre-Gaggia, pre-spring-loaded time of the 1940s. The force comes not from a powerful, heavy spring, as in the Gaggia machine, or a powerful, lightweight pump, as in the later Faema. It comes from your arm. If you don't press hard enough on the lever, the espresso won't be good. Then again, if you press too hard, it won't be good either.

The Pavoni does show clearly how crucial grind size is to successful espresso making—for professionals and home espresso makers alike, with almost any kind of machine. If the grind is too coarse, the lever of the Pavoni will go down with hardly any effort, and a whoosh of dirty water will likely overflow an espresso-sized cup. If it's too fine, you might feel your heels lifting off the ground and your forearms bulging as you try to push down the lever, listening to the steam valve hiss and threaten imminent explosion.

My family and I often experienced this anxiety as we tried to prepare perfect coffees for my espresso-loving father, to whom we gave a Pavoni one Father's Day. We made every single mistake you can make. Our experience taught us how to brew a good espresso, more or less—and that we didn't want to do it more often than on Father's Day and my father's birthday.

Solid Choices: Pump Machines

All other home espresso machines that supply proper pressure do it with pumps. Anyone can make very good espresso with a pump machine and a little practice.

Be warned that any electric pump machine makes noise—constant, loud rumbling from the pump and alarming hissing from the milk steamer. One manufacturer, Salton, tired of receiving panicked calls from customers who feared burnout or explosion, used to put stickers on its pump machines reading, "I'm noisy. I'm doing my job." Be warned, too, that the whole business of making espresso cup by cup, as pump machines require you to do, is messy. The closer you can keep the machine to a sink, the happier you'll be.

When you go shopping for a serious espresso maker, you may first be directed toward a machine that substitutes for the usual boiler a newer alternative called a thermal block. (Krups is the most familiar maker.) Even if I recognize the advantages of this newer method, I don't recommend it. In these machines, hot water spirals through a metal-alloy block, like a radiator, instead of a boiler. The machines are quieter than other pump machines and take up less counter space. The problem is that I don't find the pressure adequate.

The thermal-block machines I've seen, too, come with flimsy accoutrements. You want good, solid materials. A filter holder should feel like a hand-held weight, not like something from a child's tea-party set. The heavier the metal of the filter, filter holder and "group"—the metal housing into

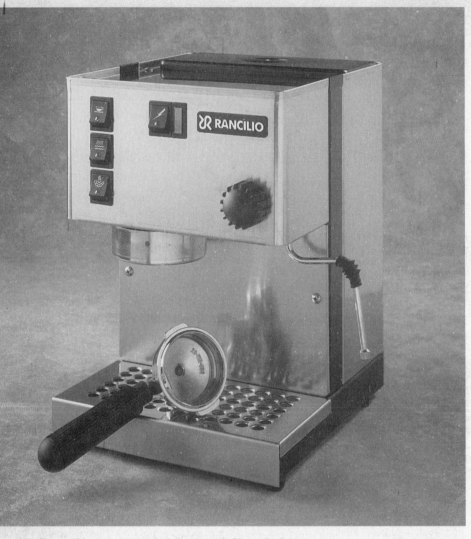

Rancilio pump machine and filter holder

which you latch the filter holder—the better they will retain heat. And a pre-heated machine is a big step toward obtaining crema.

The solidest machines are the most expensive. I keep in my kitchen a big machine by Rancilio, a maker of professional machines that also manufacturers a home line, because I know it will last forever. The boiler is brass, the most durable material, and the filter holder is interchangeable with the one in Rancilio's professional machines—of a sufficient width and heft to produce a single shot of espresso with body and crema. (Less expensive machines don't produce anything less than a double shot with success.)

I love the solidity and power of this machine, which is the closest anyone can come to a professional one without spending a few thousand dollars. The Rancilio costs about $400; other similarly solid machines cost the same and are sold by Faema and the hallowed Gaggia. These machines are tanks, utterly reliable. You still have to do a lot of wiping up, though, and you still have to get the grind just right to produce a beautiful crema. (See Using a Pump Espresso Machine, page 118.)

Lazy Solutions: Saeco and Barista

I don't use the Rancilio every day. I use a lazy person's solution to making espresso at home. It's a pump machine, marketed as Saeco or, at Starbucks, as Barista, that makes crema-covered espresso from any kind of bean, as long as the coffee is reasonably fresh. This is because the machine—a normal pump machine with a boiler, and not impressively sturdy—includes a great invention: a filter holder with a valve at the bottom. This valve means that the machine is forgiving of grind size, the toughest problem in espresso.

Brewing begins with the filter closed, which pre-infuses the grounds and also greatly increases the pressure. The loud, cranky rumbling of the pump subsides to a muffled roar after about five seconds, and you slowly open the valve by rotating the filter holder to the left. The brewed coffee is forced through a needle-sized opening at the bottom of the holder before coursing down the usual spouts.

The espresso from this filter holder is the thickest and richest of any home machine I've tried, with a lovely head of crema thanks to the presaturation, the additional pressure and the mixing of liquid with air as the coffee comes through the tiny opening. You need not worry whether the tamp is too light or too heavy or whether you've put in exactly the right amount of ground coffee—little tricks you have to learn when using other pump machines.

Machines come in several sizes. Some cost as little as $150 (if you find a good sale), although an average price is $300. I tell anyone new to espresso and eager for both convenience and the freedom to try any blend to find the cheapest model that comes with this filter holder. I also strongly recommend a flat-bottomed tamper and a "knock box," a square metal box the size of a

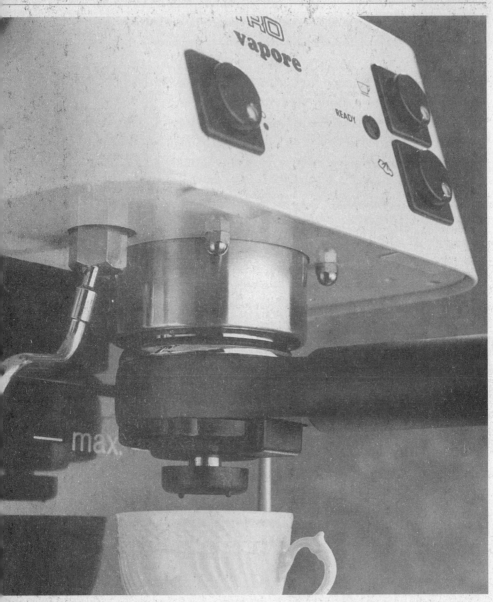

Pump machine with adjustable filter holder

largish ashtray with a rubber-coated bar mounted at the top, which makes it easy to dispose of the grounds after each cup is brewed. (The knock boxes that come with a few home machines are too flimsy.) Both the tamper and the knock box are small investments: as little as $4 for a plastic tamper and $10 to

$50 for a metal or wooden one, and about $20 to $30 for a knock box (see Sources, pages 254, 256).

Quick Fixes: Nespresso and E.S.F.

Some people don't care about experimenting with their own blends. They just want the best espresso they can get with the least trouble. I tell these people to look at machines that use prepacked doses of espresso, which fit into spe-

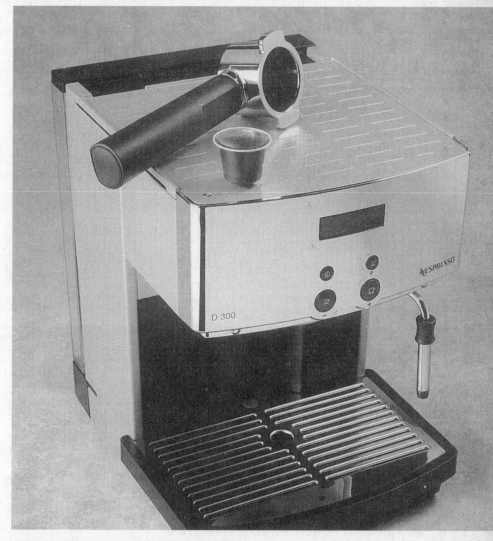

Nespresso pump machine with Nestlé capsule

cial filter holders. The first to be widely marketed were aluminum "capsules" about the shape of tiny plastic cream containers, made by Nestlé and sold for use in specially manufactured pump machines. You pop the capsule or cartridge into the filter holder, push the brew button, and that's it. The big drawback is that you're paying for a pump machine—Nespresso machines run between $200 and $650—without being able to choose your own coffee.

Another pod system, Easy Serving Espresso (E.S.E.), attempts to solve this problem by sharing a standardized design among a number of manufacturers. First developed in the 1980s by Illy, the premier Italian roaster, for use in restaurants, E.S.E. was made available for home use in 1996. Today nearly thirty companies are part of the E.S.E. consortium. Though E.S.E. pods use the same basic principle as the Nespresso cartridges, the wider selection of machines (manufacturers include Saeco, DeLonghi, Krups and FrancisFrancis!) and varieties of coffee (Illy, Lavazza and Starbucks are among the participating roasters) offer a much greater measure of flexibility. People who opt for E.S.E. need not limit themselves to prepacked espresso, either: some E.S.E.-compatible machines, like the Krups Novo 2300 and the Starbucks Barista, come with filter holders that can accommodate loose coffee or pods. Because E.S.E. pods are made of filter paper and are not airtight, they begin losing freshness as soon as the box is opened, and you should be sure to seal containers as closely as possible.

Using prepacked pods or capsules means paying a premium for convenience. Coffee costs can mount to hundreds of dollars a year for someone who drinks two or three espressos a day. Still, for anyone who isn't fond of tinkering and constant wiping, these methods are foolproof, and they offer guaranteed crema. Dozens of little turns of the wrist and considerations of how to brew the perfect espresso are unnecessary, and cleanup is simply rinsing the grounds-free filter holder and wiping the milk-steaming nozzle.

Fully Automatic

There's a last solution for people who don't want to bother with the infinite adjustments most serious espresso machines require: the soup-to-nuts, do-everything machines that take you from whole beans to drip coffee, espresso and cappuccino. I've always distrusted these machines to the point of active disapproval. It's not just the snobbery of the driver who prefers a 1967 Maserati to a Neon (or, given the price of most fully automatic machines, a BMW SUV), although there's plenty of that. Like SUVs, these machines generally take up way too much room, cost too much and, because of their clumsiness, don't work very well.

The cup for whole beans is usually impossible to empty, for example, and so the beans go stale long before you can use them up. The plastic cups collect oils that go rancid and can't be removed for thorough cleaning. The grinders themselves usually don't work very well. And that's just the grinder. Getting the ground coffee to the right chamber, running water through it at the right pressure and temperature, removing the grounds and cleaning the coffee maker—all these are fraught with the worst Rube Goldberg–contraption perils, and at a colossal price.

After trying several elephantine disasters, I gave up on the whole concept. Then a friend invited me to toy with her new Jura Impressa S90, and I became a semi-convert. Like its rich relations, the Impressa is expensive: about $1,800 retail. But unlike them, it is designed handsomely and takes up a reasonable amount of counter room for what it does—not much more than a good pump machine. The Impressa makes the error of trying to do too many things well—make drip coffee and espresso, for example—and it has as many programmable options as the most confusing DVD player.

But the Impressa does many things its predecessors did not. For example, it allows removal of the bean container and lets you put ground coffee from another source through a separate funnel to make another kind of coffee in the middle of using the beans in the main container: decaf, as the most obvious example. It also froths milk well, which most machines its size fail to.

I still prefer almost any other machine to a fully automatic—for better price, and for greater control of the many variables that lie between good and great coffee. The espressos I tried, in various quantities at a time, still had the thin texture I remember from automatic machines. But Jura is a more inventive and reliable company than most other entrants in the field, and the frother is a great improvement. For those who want to drive a Rolls (or, to make the comparison more accurate, who want to ride in the back seat of a Rolls and leave the driving to somebody else) the Impressa is a luxurious convenience.

Cappuccino and Lattes

"Yes, yes," I hear you saying. "Enough about espresso. I want to make great cappuccino and lattes." In Italy, the cappuccino, a drink named for the brown and white cowl of a Capuchin monk's habit, is the reigning milk drink. With its satiny foam, its suavely warm milk and a shot of dense, beautifully syrupy espresso, a cappuccino is indeed magisterial. The experience of cappuccino or caffè latte—an espresso drink with much more milk than a cappuccino—should be coffee mixed with hot milk, rising through a soft, liquidy layer of foam whose tiny bubbles pop as you lift the drink to your lips. All the components should blend in your mouth at once, combining sensations that slowly separate out on the palate—sweet, bitter, milky and chocolaty—not only while you swallow but afterward too.

What gives this drink its almost mystical perfection is the proportion of espresso to two kinds of heated milk, steamed and foamed. A cappuccino is classically one-third espresso, one-third steamed milk and one-third foamed milk. Steamed milk is simply milk that has been scalded—brought just to the boiling point by the injection of steam. It's hot, but its volume is unchanged. Foamed milk is both heated and aerated. It forms at the top of the milk pitcher at the end of the steaming process. The ideal consistency of foamed milk is of very lightly whipped cream that just holds its shape but is deliciously yielding.

In Italy, a caffè latte is a family drink, made in the mornings with coffee brewed in the stovetop moka and with milk heated on the stove, brought just near but never actually to the boil (this is equal to steamed milk). It's about 1 part coffee to 2 or 3 parts milk, but it can't be fairly compared to a cappuccino—the coffee is much thinner than an espresso, and the milk isn't foamed. It's more or less the same drink the French call café au lait, although because they like serving it in bowls, they put in more milk; Italians use cups the size of our teacups.

In an Italian household, you drink a caffè latte in the kitchen, barely conscious, and dunk tea biscuits right from the box. Then you go to work, and stop midmorning for a cappuccino and a *cornetto,* like a croissant but less buttery. That's more or less it for the day's coffee and milk. Every stop after that is for an espresso, drunk with sugar, or for a *caffè macchiato*—an espresso "stained" with about two tablespoons of foam. In a bar, a caffè latte is an unusual order, associated with children and convalescents, made with 1 part espresso to 4 parts steamed milk, served with no foam on top. The latte took over in this country because Americans want a longer-lasting drink than Europeans do, and it became fixed in the American coffee-bar repertory as 1 part coffee to anywhere from 3 to 8 parts steamed milk, with a crown of foam.

Steaming Wands and Steaming Machines

The way to achieve foamy nirvana is to put a pitcher of milk under a "wand," a long metal tube that delivers steam from the boiler of an espresso machine. All home espresso machines—steam, piston, pump—have a steam wand. Depending on the size of the water boiler, the steam will be weaker or stronger and longer- or shorter-lived. The biggest and most professional machines have the biggest boilers and make steaming milk easy. If your machine is on the weak side, you can buy a helpful little device to beef up the steam's effect. Or you can buy a separate machine whose boiler just makes steam for milk. You'll need one of these if you have a stovetop moka brewer, which in its classic form doesn't have a wand.

Before you buy an espresso machine, check whether the wand is movable. If it is, you'll have a simpler time positioning the pitcher and will be able to use whatever size pitcher you want. If the machine doesn't have a milk-steaming pitcher as an accessory, look for a metal pitcher whose opening is narrower than its base. An opening that is half as wide as the bottom will allow the milk to circulate and expand without spraying out. Metal will better conduct heat and retain cold, which is important because milk is easier to foam if it's cold and in a cold pitcher. Buy the size you'll need for the number of espresso drinks you're likely to make at one time—the milk will at least double in volume. A two-cup capacity is a useful size.

Many machines come with a gadget that helps make foaming easier. Usually this is a device that fits over the wand and draws air into the milk while the wand delivers steam. Without such a device, you have to keep the nozzle somewhere near the surface, so that it will both eject steam and churn air into the milk; if the nozzle is buried deep in the milk, the steam will simply heat, and not foam, the milk. With a sleeve or other such device, you can place the nozzle where you please. If your machine doesn't come with one, the

Krups Perfect Froth attachment, available at many coffee stores for about $10 (see Sources, page 254), will fit onto many nozzles. (See Foaming Milk, page 124.)

After you experiment with the wand on your machine, you might decide that you want a more powerful steamer, one whose steam won't run out just as you're getting a head of foam. This shouldn't happen with a standard pump machine, and it certainly won't happen with a Rancilio or similarly priced machine, which will have a big boiler and an efficient heater. But with electric steam-powered brewers—the kind that cost under $100—the likelihood is great that you'll run out of steam when you need it most.

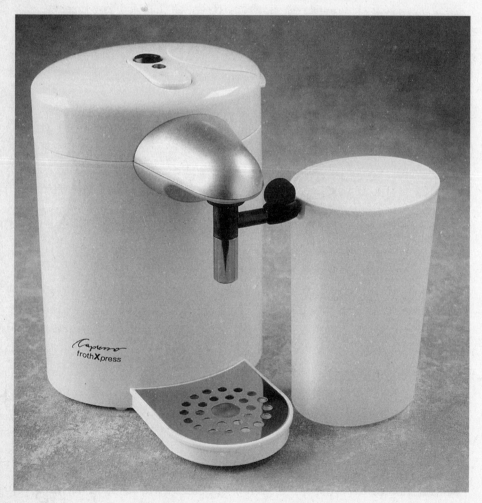

Capresso FrothXpress electric milk steamer

Electric milk steamers can come to the rescue. The machine I long recommended was the Cappuccino Crazy, made by Salton/Maxim and usually priced at about $40. This was simply a boiler connected to a tube out of which a gratifyingly strong burst of steam spurted when you pressed a lever. It was the most reliable gadget of its kind—and as this edition went to press, the manufacturer stopped making it. You can still find many examples for sale, though, on various websites.

Luckily, another company came up with its own steaming gadget. Capresso, which produces an extensive line of drip and espresso coffee makers with well-thought-out features and adjustments, makes a separate steamer, the "frothXpress." This takes the shaving cream approach, mixing hot steam, produced by a water reservoir in the back of the machine, with air and with cold milk from a separate plastic pitcher it provides. Hot foamed milk comes down a spout at the front. The great advantage, again, is reliable steamed milk in sufficient quantities for a group of guests—something no home espresso machine can provide. Also, the Capresso machine allows you to adjust the temperature of the foamed milk; the manufacturer claims possible adjustments between 120 and 170 degrees F, and pros aim for about 150 (see Foaming Milk, page 124). This is crucial for lovers of Italian cappuccino, who rightly object to the somewhat yucky taste of plain cooked milk and long for the sublime combination of sweet, creamy, foamy milk and deep, slightly bitter espresso.

Prolonging the Pleasure

Any liquid can be steamed, but foaming depends on the protein and fat that milk contains. In America, baristas have their own opinions about which milk produces the best foam. You can foam any milk, although half-and-half and cream will hardly budge after the steam heats them. Skim milk produces foam fastest, but with dry, stiff peaks that are better suited to a lemon pie or a chocolate mousse than to a cup of espresso. Dry foam is no fun to drink. It hits your lips like kapok during a pillow fight, and keeps you from getting what you want—a fragrant mixture of milk and espresso. Also, what liquid remains has been watered and seems blue. I get the best results with 1 and 2 percent milk, but that may be prejudice, because they're the kind I like most. An Italian barista would find this discussion very silly: fat is where flavor and "mouthfeel" are, and the glories of an Italian bar are built on whole milk.

Milk isn't the only way you can lengthen an espresso, which to anyone used to a full cup of coffee seems very stingy. Why not try water instead? It's a lot less fattening, and it nicely prolongs the balance and pleasure of a properly made espresso. A *caffè americano,* as an espresso elongated with hot water became known in Seattle, offers much of the balance and depth of espresso, with more to sip on. This is what espresso bars without conventional brewers offer to customers who want a full cup of "regular" coffee. (The wrong way to make this is by leaving the espresso machine on too long, which overextracts the ground coffee and throws the flavor entirely out of balance.) Espresso and water is surprisingly satisfying, and so is one of my favorite tricks—reinforcing a cup of decent but unexciting brewed coffee with a shot of espresso.

Gilding the Lily: Flavorings

You can flavor these drinks however you please, of course. Let's start with unsweetened cocoa powder and ground cinnamon, the two most common powders in canisters at bars, to be shaken over the foamed milk. The first is fine, the second verboten as far as I'm concerned. But who am I to forbid the use of an appealing spice I may love with apples but find at loggerheads with the flavors of coffee? If you like cinnamon and coffee, enjoy.

Dozens of flavored syrups that taste like orange or almond or tamarind (sourish, and very nice) or any of the other fruits and nuts for which they are named are turning up in coffee bars. Torani syrups, the most widely distributed brand, are Italian, and the multicolored labels lined up behind practically every bar in Italy make it look something like an old Wurlitzer jukebox. My stern view is that these syrups belong where the manufacturers intended them to go: in tall glasses filled with soda water, fruit juices and, often, liquor. They've caught on in coffee, though, opening a whole new market for the delighted manufacturers. So far, espresso bars don't use flavored beans, knowing that flavoring essences would be nearly impossible to clean out of the espresso machine. (Don't let flavored beans anywhere near your home espresso machine. The flavorings will contaminate every cup you brew thereafter.)

In America, just about any flavoring is considered acceptable with coffee. If you'd like to experiment, try buying one, or at most two, syrups to see how they work in your favorite drinks. I like the Monin brand, which many bars favor for its pure taste and its less distracting sugar content. Start by pouring a teaspoon into the brewed espresso. Some people put syrups into the milk pitcher along with the milk and steam the two, but I think this is a bad idea. First, you might not use all the milk, so it's hard to know just how much syrup you like in your cappuccino or latte. And flavoring essences either deteriorate or turn bitter with high heat.

I like two flavors in coffee: chocolate and vanilla. You can flavor coffee with either one in several ways besides using chocolate or vanilla syrup. For vanilla flavoring, split whole vanilla beans lengthwise (many coffee shops carry them, as well as gourmet shops) and bury them in sugar for at least a few days. This will make vanilla sugar, which will keep for months at room temperature. Sweeten your coffee with it. Or add a few drops of good-quality vanilla extract to coffee. Or sprinkle vanilla powder over black espresso or brewed coffee. The powder occasionally fills a third canister at coffee bars beside the cocoa and cinnamon, and is often sold at specialty-coffee shops.

I happen to make sensational hot cocoa, which can serve as a flavoring essence. In a saucepan, whisk together ½ cup cocoa powder, 1 teaspoon corn-starch or arrowroot, ⅓ cup sugar and ½ cup water, on or off a low flame—it will dissolve either way after thirty seconds or so. Add ½ cup more water and a cup of milk, of whatever kind you like. Keep stirring over low to moderate heat for about ten minutes, scraping the bottom to prevent scorching, until the mixture thickens.

A batch of this, using all water in place of milk, will keep for months in the refrigerator, and you can mix in a spoonful whenever you want to add chocolate flavor to something. A wonderful drink is equal parts coffee and my cocoa mixture and three parts hot milk. I think of other flavorings as gilding the lily. You may think of them as embellishing perfection.

Using a Moka

To make coffee in a stovetop moka brewer, first unscrew the base, remove the metal coffee filter and fill the bottom with cold water to the level of the safety valve. Replace the filter and spoon in enough ground coffee to reach the top. The grind should be medium-fine, about the same as for a paper filter or a little finer. If the grind is too fine, the water won't get through it, because the pressure isn't strong enough, or the water will overheat in the attempt and overextract, drawing out bitter substances. Sweep a knife edge or spatula over the top to level the coffee. You can compact the grounds slightly with the bottom of a glass that fits the diameter of the filter, but don't tamp the coffee hard or the water won't make it through.

Screw on the upper chamber and set the moka on a medium-low flame. After about three minutes, coffee will begin to hiss and dribble out two holes at the sides of the tube in the upper compartment. The tube in the upper compartment is by design partially closed, both to prevent coffee from spraying all over the stove if the lid is left open—as it generally is, so you can tell when the coffee is ready—and to add a bit more pressure to the coffee on its final journey. Some people even buy small metal caps that fit over the tube and further restrict the flow, supposedly to intensify the flavor. These don't do very much.

As soon as a dark pool collects in the bottom of the chamber and the flow of liquid changes from a slow and steady stream to a sputtering foam, turn off the heat. This will safeguard against burning the bottom of the pot. To get crema, advanced moka users fill the filter with coffee ground almost as fine as for a commercial espresso machine and tamp it before brewing. This might intensify the flavor, but I don't recommend it, because you run the risk of burning out the rubber gasket.

If you simply leave the top open and lower the flame about midway through, you can obtain espresso better than many people ever get in their electric steam espresso or even their pump espresso machines. Don't get hung up on producing crema. If you do get any, think of it as some astral blessing.

Using a Pump Espresso Machine

Here are useful steps that apply to just about every home pump espresso machine. You should, of course, first read the instruction manual, because each machine has different features.

As with any electric brewer, the first step is to clean out the dust by running water through the machine without any coffee. You'll repeat this "blind" brewing whenever you use the machine, in order to heat all the metal parts and the cups too. Running several 8-ounce cups of water through the machine the first time, into a bowl or measuring cup, will also show you how quickly the removable water reservoir empties and give you an idea of how often you'll have to replenish it. Refilling the reservoir is crucial if you want to avoid burning out the pump—something that would necessitate expensive repairs.

Whenever you brew, first prime the pump, which will freshen the water in the boiler and flush out any stray air pockets. You can do this by pressing the espresso-brewing button or by opening the nozzle on the steam wand—a faster way to get water circulating but a messy one, since without some kind of cup or pitcher under the nozzle, or a towel wrapped around it, it will spray water onto you and the counter. Water will pour out the "shower head," as the diffuser screen in the metal housing for the filter holder is aptly called; set a bowl under it. (If you can't put the machine next to the sink, you'll also want a bowl nearby to hold the excess water.) Stop running the water and wait for the light to indicate that the water is hot enough to brew coffee. Run hot water through the empty filter holder into the serving cup or cups just before loading the filter holder and brewing.

This seemingly endless running of water might sound wasteful, but hot *everything* is essential. In fact it's a good idea to dump the first cup of brewed espresso. The second cup will always taste better, and especially if you're allowing yourself only one cup, it should be as good as you can make it. Logically that would mean using bottled water, too, but you'll have to dump so much water while heating everything that it would be not only wasteful but expensive. Water from a filter pitcher (see Sources, page 253) is a cheaper alternative.

Because the correct grind size is vital, using beans professionally ground for electric home espresso machines, preferably from a careful coffee shop, will make experimenting easier. If you buy ground coffee in a can or vacuum pack, the label should clearly state that the grind is for espresso only—"all-purpose" grinds are rarely good for any purpose at all. When you rub the coffee between your fingers it should feel like fine sand, with something of an abrasive grit. You should not feel the flannel softness of flour, which will clog up the works.

Loading and Latching

Use the scoop supplied with the machine to measure the coffee into the preheated filter. Most machines come with single and double filters, but I recommend using only the double filter. Small quantities just don't come out right in home machines, unless you buy one of the few that use professional-sized filter holders, which are much wider and provide a bed adequate to hold and diffuse the water. The scoop should hold 6.5 to 7 grams of ground coffee, roughly ¼ ounce. This is about 2 tablespoons, about the same as a standard brewing scoop.

Don't worry too much about measurements. Espresso brewing requires far more improvisation than filtered coffee, because of the variables of equipment and weather. More important than precise measurement is the grind size, how finely you compact the ground coffee with the tamping tool provided, and whether or not you leave headroom in the filter for the grounds to expand once they're wet. Too big a "dose," as the Italians call the measure of coffee that goes into the filter, and you'll have trouble latching the filter holder securely into the metal housing; the grounds won't be able to expand properly, holding up the flow of water and resulting in unevenly extracted espresso.

The purpose of tamping is to level the surface of the ground coffee in the filter and compact it, providing an evenly resistant bed for the stream of water. Don't overdo it. Too much tamping and the water won't make it through the coffee, and you'll hear increasingly loud rumbling as the pump keeps trying. If you don't tamp at all, though, the water might go through the ground coffee too fast and underextract the coffee.

The tamper should be slightly narrower than the filter and have a flat bottom. Many manufacturers dumbly include tampers with convex bottoms —relics of a time long gone when filter bottoms were convex too. Using such a tamper with today's filters will likely throw off the extraction: the water will go through the middle too fast relative to the higher sides. Buy a flat-bottomed tamper or hunt for a cup or glass whose base will fit neatly into the filter. Make sure the base is dry, so coffee won't stick to it. Press the tamper down firmly, and if you want to get into the spirit of things, twist the tamper a quarter turn to "polish" the ground coffee. Wipe any stray ground coffee— there will be some—off the rim of the filter holder so as not to interfere with the seal of the machine.

The filter holder should be firmly latched into the machine, which generally means a half turn. It's easy to do this wrong, especially if you've overloaded the filter. The holder can remain in place but not be secure. (While fooling with unfamiliar machines, I several times watched the filter holder crash into the cup when I turned on the water.) The simplest way to be certain is to bend down and check that the handle of the filter holder is parallel to the counter. If you have problems latching in the holder, bend down again and peer into the inner surface of the metal housing, which might well be blocked by old coffee grounds. A flexible brush like a pipe cleaner will help clear them out.

Brewing

Be sure the brew light indicates that the water is hot enough for brewing. This might take a minute if you've been careful to brew blind beforehand, heating up the metal housing and the filter holder. Don't forget to heat the cup itself, either by leaving it under the filter holder to catch hot water when brewing blind or by simply rinsing it with hot tap water. Or you can keep the cups in a pot of very hot water, as baristas in Naples do, using forceps to remove them. (Take the pot off the stove before you put in the cups, and be sure the cups are sturdy.) Heavy ceramic cups will best retain heat, and demitasse cups will best display the perfume of espresso.

Although you can't regulate the pressure, you can use a few barista tricks to get the most from your machine. One is to pre-infuse the ground coffee in the filter by letting water flow into it for just a second or two. This means pressing the brew button quickly and then switching it off. The hot water will expand the grounds and make them more evenly resistant to the water that then comes through, just as with manual drip brewing. Many fancy computerized professional machines are programmed to do this automatically (spring-loaded piston machines do it too). Then you press the brew button again and wait for espresso to start flowing into the cup.

Most shots brewed in a home machine are at their best in a much shorter time than their instructions would have it—usually fifteen seconds rather than twenty-five to thirty. As with the exact dose of coffee you use, this is more a matter of judging by eye and experience than adhering to a precise rule. The ideal flow of espresso begins thick, slow and in a gently curving steady black drip, like honey from a spoon (Italians call it a *coda di topo*, or "mouse tail"). After five or ten seconds, it turns to a pour. Air begins to enter and the color lightens.

Then, if you're lucky, crema comes out, with very fine bubbles and a warm straw color. This golden moment is brief. As soon as large bubbles appear on the surface, snatch the cups from under the filter—*do not* let the last dribs and drabs enter the cup after you shut off the water.

Never brew espresso for longer than it takes to make 1½ liquid ounces per shot. You'll get all kinds of unpleasant substances you don't want to taste if you do. You defeat all the care you take and the money you spend if you overextract espresso, and the easiest way to do that is to brew it too long. Perfection lies in knowing when to stop.

No Crema? What Went Wrong

Specialists diagnose espresso by the color and amount of crema that appears. First, you won't get crema at all if the beans aren't fresh, and in a home machine, the sad fact is that you'll have trouble getting it, period. But achieving crema is by no means impossible. The ideal is a layer about ⅛ inch thick that remains on the cup for at least thirty seconds or a minute—by which time you should have downed the espresso—and that will hold ½ teaspoon of sugar on the surface before letting it sink gently to the bottom of the cup.

If the color is just off-white and the layer of crema dissipates quickly, the espresso is underextracted. The remedies include making sure the water and everything it passes through are hot; grinding the beans a notch finer and making sure the dose is large enough; tamping harder and stopping the brew sooner. Stop brewing as soon as the bubbles in the crema go from looking like a very fine sea spray to a messier one, with bubbles you can actually detect on the surface.

If the crema is dark and burnt-looking, the espresso probably will taste burnt too. Other signs of overextraction are a hole or a dark spot in the middle. Remedies include setting the grinder a bit coarser, being sure to leave enough headroom in the filter, easing up on both the dose and the tamping, and cutting off the water sooner.

If the drips are a long time coming and never turn into a pour, or you don't get any drips at all and the rumbling of the pump is abnormally loud, then the grind is too fine, you've added too much ground coffee, or you've tamped it too hard. Remove the filter holder—slowly, since there might be a good deal of built-up pressure above it—and press the brew button to be sure that water is still coming out of the shower head. If no water comes out, be sure the reservoir is full, and open the control for the steam wand to get water circulating. Wipe off the shower head to try to clear out any grounds that may be clogging it. This is also a good step to take if plain hot water comes out the sides of the filter head just as espresso is flowing out the bottom—usually a sign of a dirty or deformed gasket around the shower head, and a very common problem. To avoid deforming the gasket, don't leave the spent grounds in the latched-in holder.

In general, you stand a much better chance of producing crema with beans that are unwashed, that is, dry-processed, before they are roasted —a piece of information you rarely get at a specialty-coffee shop. Many African and some Indonesian and South American arabica beans are un-washed. Washing seems to remove protective oils that help greatly in the formation of colloids, which form crema. Almost any robusta bean is un-washed, and so robusta in an espresso blend is pretty much a guaranteed crema-producer, even though careful drinkers object to its deadening flavor. The way to taste for yourself is to buy a can of inexpensive Italian coffee, which is sure to contain a high percentage of robusta. Unwashed arabicas—in Italian blends, typically Brazilian beans—and robustas will also produce stronger body, which will help carry through milk in a coffee-milk drink.

Whether or not you see crema emerging, cut off the water at 2½ ounces—less than a ¼-cup measure—for a double shot. If you don't have a measuring cup in liquid ounces that will fit under the filter holder, look for a couple of shot glasses at the hardware store and measure their capacity, which will be anywhere from 1 to 3 ounces. Set the shot glasses under the filter holder instead of cups.

Cleaning the Filter Holder

Each time you make a new espresso, you'll have to empty and rinse the filter holder. Wait a bit between shots, or accumulated pressure above the holder might spurt coffee mud when you take it out. This isn't a problem when using a thermal-block machine, which doesn't retain pressure, or an expen-sive pump machine with a boiler, which will have a helpful feature called a "backflush" tube.

Where to dump the grounds? Knocking the full filter holder against the side of a garbage or compost can or the edge of a sink-mounted disposer

—the usual solutions—can result in a bashed-in holder or a lost filter (the filter holders supplied with some home machines have little latches to keep the filter from falling out). A separate knock box is a worthwhile, small investment. You whack the filter squarely across the middle and smartly rap out the spent grounds. If you don't have a knock box, use a spoon to dig out the grounds.

Never use steel wool or any kind of abrasive detergent on the filter or holder, which can become scratched and collect coffee oils that will turn rancid. Many baristas don't believe in using any soap at all, fearing that it will impart off flavors to the coffee. Instead they soak the filter and holder in a solution with a special powdered detergent made for coffee equipment. You occasionally find these powders, with names like Puly Caff and Puro Caff, in specialty stores, or you can mail-order them. Professionals run detergent solutions like these through their machines—something you should do, too, but only if the directions for the machine recommend it. Special detergent or not, it's a good idea to soak the filter and filter holder overnight, to work grounds out of the bottom of the filter and remove stains from the holder.

The irritating fact is that in making espresso carefully you need to spend more time cleaning than brewing. Every few times you brew, wipe out the group and try to scrub the shower head, so grounds won't clog it. Darker roasts are oilier, so if you're using them for espresso, as is likely, you'll have to be especially vigilant with the scrub brush. The messiest part of all is likely to be the drip tray at the bottom of the machine, where sludge collects. It's the part easiest to forget to clean, since it's usually covered by a screen.

Foaming Milk

Just as everything should be hot in brewing espresso, everything should be cold in foaming milk. A metal pitcher is quickly chilled in the refrigerator or freezer, which will ease the incorporation of air. In a pinch, you can use a mug or cup. If you have a ready supply of ice cubes, you can stash a heatproof metal or glass container in ice for a few minutes while the machine heats.

The time a home machine takes between heating water for coffee and "superheating" water for steam (to as high as 239 degrees F) is called the dwell time, and it can be frustratingly long—longer even than the machine shows it to be. If you open the steam wand as soon as the light indicates that the water is hot enough, you'll likely be greeted by a piddling trickle of hot water. The light is a measurement of temperature, not pressure. To build up pressure and get more reliable steam, leave the machine on for a few minutes after the light says it's ready.

Because the wait is so long, I think it's better to foam milk before brewing espresso. Heated milk can withstand a minute or two's wait far better than espresso can. If need be, you can always fluff it back up just before pouring it into the espresso. Once the milk is cold and thoroughly deflated, though, you cannot successfully refoam it, no matter how hard you try; it contains too much condensed water.

Before you begin, be sure to blow out any leftover water in the tubes by opening the steam valve into an empty container or a towel (double or triple the towel so you don't burn yourself). Fill the container one-third full. The bigger the container, the easier it is to foam milk: aim for a 2-cup container so that you can practice on 1 cup milk. Assuming you have a naked nozzle without any kind of sleeve or foam-enhancing attachment, place it just under the surface of the milk.

You want steady but not overwhelming steam. If you open the valve all the way, the surface of the milk will look like it's in the middle of a hurricane. The desired effect is of a motorboat engine creating a discreet rather than a wild wake, or a Jacuzzi that makes the surface of bathwater look like twined rope. If the surface is becalmed and the noise stifled, move up the nozzle. If the surface heaves violently and big bubbles form, move the nozzle deeper into the liquid and turn down the steam a little. Sound will be your chief guide. Try to keep the motion of the pitcher smooth and slow.

A few seconds too long can be disastrous, as with espresso. You'll overheat the milk, and it will have that yucky cooked-milk taste. The simplest rule is that if a metal pitcher is too hot to hold comfortably, the milk will be too hot and will taste bad. A more scientific way to check is to buy a thermometer that clips to the side of the pitcher; steam until the thermometer reads anywhere from 135 to 150 degrees F. You're aiming for a final temperature of 150 to 170 degrees, but if you wait until the thermometer gives that reading, the milk will continue to heat while you crank down the steam. After a few tries, you'll know where to stop with your own steamer. If you boil the milk by mistake, throw it away.

Look for small, even bubbles rather than big ones, which, like those in crema at the top of espresso, will dissipate fast. The goal is not a hearty head of foam, as on a mug of beer, but aerated milk with a velvety texture. Don't despair if you get bubbly foam instead of fine foam: as long as you haven't overheated the milk, you can rap the pitcher against the counter to knock out the excess air. While you brew the espresso, the consistency of the milk will settle into something like the stable foam you seek.

Wipe the nozzle each and every time after you steam milk. Dried coffee grounds and rancid oils are nothing compared with caked-on milk, which adheres to the nozzle like enamel. If you forget to wipe the nozzle and milk does cake on, use a scouring pad and plenty of elbow grease—not an abrasive cleanser, which will pit the metal parts—to vanquish it. Or let time do the work and submerge the nozzle in a glass of room-temperature or hot water for a couple of hours. The tiny holes at the end of the nozzle often clog too. While the nozzle is still hot and there's still steam, blast some through the holes to be sure they're clear. If you don't have time to do that, try cleaning out the holes with a safety pin or a needle.

After foaming milk and before brewing espresso, run an espresso-sized cup or two of water through the empty filter holder before charging it with ground coffee to avoid scalding it. This will vent the very hot water left over from steam production and, as a benefit, heat everything, which will encourage nice crema as you brew. Then you're ready to assemble a really fresh drink.

Making a Caffè Macchiato, Cappuccino or Caffè Latte

Find a slope-sided cup or bowl to serve the drink in, preferably one that comfortably holds 6 ounces but not much more. If you try to sip a milk-based coffee drink from a straight-sided cup, you're likely to get a mouthful of air and a fat white mustache.

Steam the milk, aiming for a warm, liquidy combination of milk and foam that is a bit under twice the volume of the milk you started with. Then brew the espresso, making sure the cup is hot. Give the milk a little more steam if it has begun to deflate. If the top seems to have dried, stir some milk back into it.

For a caffè macchiato, dot the surface of an espresso, in the usual small cup, with just a tablespoon or two of the milk, aiming to leave a brown ring visible around the edges.

For a cappuccino, pour *no more than ½ cup milk* over the waiting espresso. (This is more milk than an Italian would use—the Italian measure would be ¼ to ⅓ cup milk—but it's the minimum amount most Americans enjoy.) Ideally, this will be ¼ cup steamed milk and ¼ cup foam, and the foam will spread pertly over the surface, holding its shape just enough to leave visible a brown rim around the edge. Use a large spoon to block the foam at first so that hot milk comes out, and then to spread the foam over the top.

As for a caffè latte, if you make one according to Italian standards, it is 1 part espresso to 4 parts steamed milk, with no foam on top. What is called a caffè latte in America is really a giant-sized cappuccino, because it generally has a head of foam. The proportion is 1 part coffee to 4 or 6 or even 8 parts milk, with one or more of the parts of milk being foam. The best thing to do at home is decide how much milk and foam you like to how much coffee, and then call the drink whatever you like.

Espresso at a Glance

Stovetop Moka

ADVANTAGES: Easy, convenient, low-tech, cheap. Makes several cups at a time. Coupled with a separate milk steamer, provides the cheapest alternative for making cappuccino and caffè latte.

DISADVANTAGES: Does not produce true espresso; only the greater pressure from a pump or piston machine gives espresso's thick texture and intense flavor.

LOOK FOR: Stainless-steel versions of the familiar faceted aluminum pots with cinched waists; aluminum reacts with the acids in coffee.

BUY: Spare gaskets.

GRIND: Medium-fine.

BREW TIPS: Fill the metal basket for the coffee to the top and level off with a knife—do not tamp hard, or the water won't make it through. Leave the top open so you can see when the coffee starts pouring out the center tube; when the flow turns to sputtering foam, turn off the heat to avoid burning the bottom of the pot.

Electric Steam-Powered Machine

ADVANTAGES: Makes several cups at a time. Less temperamental than the more expensive pump machine, and more forgiving of errors in grind.

DISADVANTAGES: An expensive way to produce coffee of the same quality as stovetop pots—which is to say, it does not make true espresso. Accoutrements are usually flimsy. A milk-steaming wand rarely supplies enough pressure to steam even a small pitcher of milk.

LOOK FOR: A machine that allows you to stop brewing when you want to, so that you can obtain more powerful coffee; many machines require you to brew a full pot at a time.

BUY: A steam-enhancement gadget like the Krups Perfect Froth to help along the generally weak steamer.

GRIND: Medium-fine to fine.

BREW TIPS: When using a machine that allows you to stop brewing, cut short the brew cycle somewhere after the midway point.

Home Piston Machine (The Pavoni)

ADVANTAGES: Great looks.

DISADVANTAGES: Very expensive. Hard to operate. Inconsistent results are the rule: success depends on the proper fine grind and when and how fast you raise and push down the lever.

BUY: A high-quality burr grinder or coffee ground commercially for espresso machines.

GRIND: Fine.

BREW TIPS: Don't wait too long to lift the lever after the light indicates that the machine is ready to brew, or you'll have trouble pushing it back down.

Pump Machine

ADVANTAGES: Supplies sufficient pressure to rival coffee-bar espresso. Aside from capsule and cartridge machines (which are also powered by pumps), these are the only way to get real espresso at home. And unlike the other machines, these allow you to use any kind of coffee you like.

DISADVANTAGES: Expensive. Noisy. Each model has its own required little tricks to produce the best coffee. Very sensitive to grind size. Messy to use. Requires cleanup and reheating of accoutrements for each one or two cups. If the boiler is small, steam pressure for steaming milk can fizzle out when you most need it.

LOOK FOR: Very heavy-feeling accoutrements (filter holder, metal filter). Adjustable steam wand instead of a wand that is fixed in one position. Large-capacity water reservoir and boiler.

BUY: A flat-bottomed tamper if the tamper supplied with the machine has a convex bottom. A "knock box" for neat disposal of coffee grounds. A high-quality burr grinder or coffee ground commercially for espresso machines.

GRIND: Fine.

BREW TIPS: Run hot water through every metal part that will come into contact with the coffee before loading the filter and brewing each cup. Throw out the first cup—the second cup will always taste better. If making a milk drink, such as cappuccino or caffè latte, foam the milk first, run hot water through the filter holder to preheat it and, lastly, brew the espresso.

Pump Machine with Adjustable Filter Holder (Saeco and Barista)

ADVANTAGES: Filter holders increase the pressure of the hot water through the ground coffee, making potent espresso with guaranteed crema. Far less sensitive to grind than other pump machines.

DISADVANTAGES: Not available for the solidest machines, which produce steam for milk more reliably.

LOOK FOR: Adjustable steam wand.

GRIND: Medium-fine to fine.

BREW TIPS: Leave a fair amount of headroom in filter. Don't tamp the coffee too hard.

Pump Machine with Prepacked Ground Coffee (Nespresso and E.S.E.)

ADVANTAGES: Foolproof. You need not worry about correct grind size or cleanup.

DISADVANTAGES: You're paying full price for a pump machine, but you can't use any coffee other than the manufacturer's. Restocking capsules and cartridges can run into big money, depending on how much espresso you drink.

Milk Steamer

ADVANTAGES: Boiler is dedicated to producing steam for milk alone, meaning you'll have steady and forceful steam—something none but the most expensive pump machines offer.

DISADVANTAGES: Stovetop models may not release steam efficiently if the valve is designed poorly. No machine warns you when the boiler is about to run dry, but this is rarely a problem unless you foam quarts of milk at a time.

LOOK FOR: Electric machines, such as the Capresso frothXpress, which will spare you worry over achieving enough pressure.

BUY: Metal pitchers that slope inward in the correct size (not too big) for the amount of milk you generally foam. A nonabrasive scouring pad, to clean the milk off the wand after each use.

TIPS: Be sure the milk and the pitcher are very cold. Keep steam coming at a slow and steady rate, to avoid producing bubble-bath foam that will quickly deflate.

7 | Coffee by Country

CHAPTER SEVEN

W ALKING INTO A SHOP that sells coffee beans can be like visiting a supermarket in a foreign country. You're surrounded by things that look familiar, but you're not sure how they'll taste or how to ask for what you want. The names of the beans the store sells are rarely of immediate help either. Is Colombia Excelso the most exalted form of a famous bean, which must be great because Colombian coffee is so heavily advertised? Is Kenya AA better than plain Kenya, and how are beans from Kenya and Colombia different? Is Bourbon Santos the name of a country, a region, a kind of bean? What does the Mandheling in Sumatra Mandheling mean—is it a grade, a place, a variety?

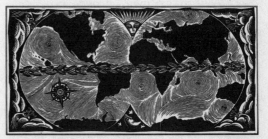

Probably the best example of the confusion behind names is the seemingly straightforward Mocha-Java blend. "Mocha" originally referred to beans shipped from the port of Mocha (Al Mukha in Arabic), on the Arabian Peninsula in the country now called Yemen. Here, just across the Red Sea from Ethiopia, where coffee trees grew wild, coffee was first cultivated and commercialized. Because these were the first beans made popular in Europe, "Mocha" became synonymous with coffee, and when chocolate arrived in Europe from the New World, it was thought to be similar in taste.

Today beans from Yemen—the only ones that can truly be called Mocha beans—are extremely rare, and they don't taste like chocolate. Nor do they even pass through Al Mukha: over a hundred years ago, the port was blocked by a sandbar. But "mocha" lives on, to describe anything with the combination of coffee and chocolate and also as part of the first and still most famous coffee blend.

Mocha-Java at a supermarket or coffee shop seldom contains a single bean of either true Mocha or Java coffees. Java, of course, is still a real place—one of the main islands of Indonesia, which the Dutch colonized and made a center of coffee production. So successful were they that "Java" has remained slang for coffee. But today the beans of Java are often considered too expensive in relation to their quality, and so roasters use just about anything they feel like in the blend.

Someone experienced in the coffee business does have a sense of how a Mocha-Java blend should taste, because he or she has tasted the wild, winy beans of Yemen and the full-bodied, earthy beans of Indonesia. So the name does carry some meaning. Most other blend names, though, like Dancing Goats blend and Rachel's Favorite, are deliberately opaque. Blends are a roaster's signature—the flavor that will keep people coming back—and are proprietary. Comparison shopping is possible for Kenya AAs, say, but not for one Dancing Goats over another.

Also, a bean menu is a moving target, because coffee is seasonal. Depending on when and how often a country harvests its coffee trees, and the political conditions there, certain beans will be available in some months and not others. Blends are constants: by perfecting his or her own, a roaster can bypass the problems of spotty availability, learning which bean can be substituted for another with as little difference in taste as possible. The beans of an entire country, by contrast, can vanish from a menu for months or even years.

In the absence of much enlightening information, customers usually judge beans by how dark they are or whether they are pretty and evenly shaped. The appearance of roasted beans, though, tells very little about how they will taste. Color does give an idea of whether acids will lend their sparkle, as they do in a medium-light roast with no oil or very little oil on the surface, or whether a full-bodied, bittersweet but possibly bland flavor will dominate, as in a heavy roast with oil on the surface. And fragmented beans can be a sign of poor handling after picking and during shipment, which often implies taste defects, or careless handling in the roasting plant, which usually doesn't. Beyond these very rough guidelines, you can't predict how a roasted bean will taste by looking at it.

No wonder most coffee customers stick to one kind of bean or blend—often one they were able to taste brewed in the store. But it's not so hard to teach yourself about the beans of the world, especially if you can find an enthusiastic coffee seller who will help you identify what makes you happiest in a "straight" bean or in a blend. Try to familiarize yourself with at least one coffee from each of the main growing areas I'll describe, and then zero in on your favorites—which, once you're used to them, you might even try blending on your own.

Be prepared to taste something different every time you buy a bag of beans, even if the label says the same thing that it did before. Flavors change with every roast. And don't stay wedded to one coffee. Taste and quality vary with each crop and each shipment.

Sorting by Region

The most sensible way to think about the countries that grow coffee is to sort them into the world's principal coffee-growing regions: Africa, Indonesia and Central and South America. As a very general rule, coffees grown near each other have similar traits. If a particular bean is unavailable, a buyer making up a blend will usually look to the country next door. "I want to start with a Central," a blender will say, meaning one of the delicate, sparkling beans grown in Central America, or "Let's make this interesting with an Africa," land of wild-tasting beans, or "The anchor will be an Indonesia," since no other beans have such powerful, mouth-filling body.

I'll take up the regions in the order in which coffee played an important role. Coffee trees first grew in Africa, and they were first cultivated in the fourteenth century by Arab colonists both in eastern Africa and on the nearby

Arabian Peninsula. The Dutch broke the commercial monopoly that had been established by Turkish merchants, bringing coffee trees from the Malabar Coast of India to their colonies in Indonesia, where they established plantations that came to dominate world coffee trade during the eighteenth century. Early in that century, one lone tree crossed the Atlantic Ocean to the Caribbean, in a hemisphere where coffee had never grown. By the end of the 1800s, little more than a century later, Central and South America had achieved their current preeminence.

Beans taste different depending on where they grow. What determines flavor is the species and variety of coffee tree, the kind of soil it grows in, the climate and altitude of the plantation, the care with which the fruit is picked, and how the beans, or seeds, are processed. All these factors vary by region, and roasters and blenders look for regional characteristics to give a signature flavor to a blend. You can look for them, too, in pursuit of your dream coffee.

An exhaustive coffee atlas is of little help, because so many countries export beans of minor or no interest—the kind that end up in a can on a supermarket shelf. Most of these would be plain boring to drink, despite the romantic and exotic sound of their names (Peru, Santo Domingo, Bahia, Ecuador; Vietnam has fast become a coffee colossus, but so far it is noted more for its enterprise than the quality of its low-growing beans). At best, these coffees are neutral, providing a calming balance for beans that could be almost too exciting on their own and serving as glue to keep everything together. Within each region, I'll discuss the countries in order of how highly their beans are valued by connoisseurs.

I'll discuss only arabica beans. Specialty roasters usually sell only these, since arabicas are the beans of highest quality—in fact, they are what separates specialty from mass-market coffee. Discussing only arabica beans eliminates many countries, such as Angola, Congo and Zaire, which grow almost exclusively robusta beans—the low-grown, cheap kind that usually taste more like a paper bag than anything else. If you've ever tasted coffee brewed from what came out of a supermarket can, you've tasted robusta, which makes up the great majority of just about every big company's house coffee.

Decoding the Lingo

It's not so hard to make things easier for the bean innocent who eagerly goes to a shop for some fine coffee. But you wouldn't know it judging by a typical coffee menu. The names of beans frequently include impressive-sounding but meaningless grading terms, which are of far more value to professional coffee buyers than to civilian coffee consumers.

Merchants should save their precision for describing where the beans were grown and how they were processed. Far more helpful than exotic or whimsical names or obscure grading terms is to group coffees by the three principal regions, and to indicate at which altitude the coffee grew. The higher the growing region, according to rule of thumb, the more delicate the flavor and the crisper the acidity.

A straightforward country name, including first country and then region within it, will mean more than any of the coffee-lingo terms that are so often thrown in. For instance, "peaberry" sometimes appears at the end of a bean name, as if to indicate something special. A peaberry is simply a common botanical peculiarity—a single rather than a double bean inside the coffee fruit, round-bellied rather than flat on one side. Some people think that pea-berries have better flavor, and others don't. The Spanish word for peaberry, *caracol*, is sometimes used, which sounds confusingly like a region or country. Another term for a botanical peculiarity, "Maragogipe," is both a region, in the Bahia section of Brazil, and the name of a variety. But its use in the trade is for a size—this time jumbo—and it usually has even less bearing on flavor. Any country can grow a Maragogipe cross with a local variety.

Other grading terms like "excelso" and "supremo" sound like they directly affect quality, when they have nothing to do with it—they just mean size. But they sound good, so merchants put them in the name. "Strictly hard bean" does have some meaning for quality: it usually refers to beans grown at the highest altitude, where a cooler climate slows growth, making beans harder and denser and intensifying flavor. Again, though, the term won't be of much help on a list of beans, because its sound-alike, "hard bean," meaning a lower grade, is often used, too, and "hard bean" rarely signifies a coffee of particular interest.

One piece of information is unexpectedly important: whether the beans were washed or dry-processed before being shipped. This may sound obscure, but aside from whether a bean is arabica or robusta and where it came from, probably no other piece of information better predicts flavor in the cup. "Washed" and "naturals" occupy separate kingdoms. The great majority of beans a specialty merchant sells have been washed, which is the more careful and expensive way of processing. This means that they not only look but taste clean: the flavors sing through, especially the lively, brightening acids. The tradeoff is a loss of body—mouth-filling viscosity that adds mightily to an enjoyable cup—and of the wild, gamy flavors that can develop when coffee cherries are left to dry in the sun.

Yemen and Ethiopia: Overarching Wildness

The supreme example of wild tastes in dry-processed beans is a true Mocha, from Yemen, and similar beans from the Harrar and Djimmah regions of Ethiopia, facing Yemen across the narrow Red Sea. The majority are still harvested from cultivars of ancient varieties. Because of the name recognition Mocha commands, all these beans are often marketed as "Mocha." For a connoisseur, each bean is different, but for a neophyte, the beans are importantly alike—and exciting. The overarching taste is of wildness, making Mochas and Harrars fruity and winy, like no other coffee.

Beans from Mattari and Sanani, two of Yemen's four growing regions, are the commonest of the true Mochas that are exported. If a shop goes to the expense of buying a real Mocha, it will usually put one of the two names on the label. Connoisseurs discuss the distinctions between them: Mattari can have more body, chocolate flavor notes and acidity; Sanani can be wilder and more aromatic, and stand up to a darker roast. These distinctions might well be too fine for anyone to worry about, as Mary Williams, who buys green coffee for Starbucks and constantly travels to producing countries, points out, because supplies are so scarce. Also, most good beans are shipped into and out of the port of Hodeida, in northern Yemen. Exporters, she says, can just slap one of the two names on a bag depending on what a broker ordered.

If the Mocha you buy is really from Ethiopia, it will likely be one of two dry-processed Ethiopians, Harrar and Djimmah. Harrar is by far the more sought after, for what Williams calls its "blueberry" flavor. Even if you find only Djimmah (which is usually processed less carefully and is therefore less highly regarded), you should buy some, because nothing matches the gamy excitement of a good dry-processed coffee. The surest sign of authenticity for any of these beans is a high price: all are rare. As with all wild foods, you're taking a chance. Genuine Harrar is quite variable, as are many dry-processed beans. Sometimes the wildness can border on dirty, and the fruity notes can vanish.

Not all beans from Ethiopia are dry-processed. When coffee people think of Ethiopia, they think fondly of the Sidamo growing region, where coffees are generally, but not always, washed. This allows more delicate flavors to show through: lemony and flowery notes, with a kind of perfumed scent and taste found only in Ethiopian beans. Some people even taste tealike flavors in Sidamo coffees. A smaller and higher area within Sidamo called Yergacheffe produces the most fragrant Sidamos (a bag will usually say either Sidamo or Ethiopian Yergacheffe). These floral and perfumed notes might be a part of the original coffee experience. So is the exciting gaminess of dry-processed beans.

Kenya: Sparkling Acidity

Aside from the wild-card coffees of Yemen and Ethiopia, most arabica beans from Africa are washed, and of the continent's washed arabicas, those of Kenya are wondrous, according to their loyal fans—higher in sparkling acidity than any beans in the world except those from Costa Rica and Guatemala. Altitude certainly helps explain the superiority of Kenyan beans. Kenya has exceedingly high coffee-growing plains—five-thousand-foot plateaus not far from Nairobi, in the foothills of Mount Kenya. (Only Peru grows beans higher, and they are seldom noteworthy.)

Farmers in Kenya have improved upon traditions begun by the German tradesmen and British colonialists who launched Kenya's coffee industry, and Kenya's concern for quality ensures, on average, the purest and most balanced cup available from African beans. The sorting, washing and preparation of beans is of a sophistication matched only in Costa Rica, Colombia and a few other countries that have, like Kenya, put government support behind the coffee trade. In a grading system unique to Kenya, the biggest beans are graded AA, one of seven rankings by size, shape and density; this is another designation that may or may not mean something in the cup. AA+ beans— usually signifying extraordinary estate-grown coffees—can fetch twice the price of AA, even if they're so scarce that you'll rarely see the term on a bag.

George Howell, founder of the East Coast chain The Coffee Connection and the new Copacafé, made Kenya a personal obsession for at least a decade, traveling frequently to meet farmers and offering a cash prize to improve the country's already high standards of processing. For his Kenyas, Howell would go through sample after sample, looking for beans that have what he calls "blackberry" flavor—a taste like a sharply acidic, only slightly sweet berry. Other merchants, too, are sometimes lucky enough to find this quality in the samples they order. Even if not every Kenya is guaranteed to be great, it's hard to go wrong by picking one, as is the case with Costa Rican coffee.

No other African country inspires the loyalty and enthusiasm of Ethiopia and Kenya, but Burundi, Malawi, Tanzania and Zimbabwe all produce arabicas that can be noteworthy. Tanzanian coffees closely resemble the more ordinary Kenyas; good ones have a winy acidity. Burundi's arabicas can be both bright in acidity and full-bodied, and therefore useful in blends; at their best they rival good Ethiopian beans. Specialty merchants offer Zimbabwes alone after a good harvest, for their acidity and hints of black pepper along with medium body; in other years, Zimbabwes will be relegated to blends. In a similar and somewhat lower tier, depending on the harvest, fall the washed arabicas of Zambia and of Uganda and Zaire (now the Democratic Republic of Congo), which grow arabicas in the Ruwenzori Mountains on their shared border.

Political difficulties in most of these countries make quality and availability uncertain from year to year. News of a washed-out bridge on the main route to a processing factory during harvest can threaten a whole season's supply. Civil wars—in Ethiopia and Rwanda, to take recent examples—can make coffees vanish for years at a time, bringing yet more misery to countries that rely on the income coffee generates. And the vagaries of climate can mean that a coffee will not live up to an initial impression from season to season. The enormous variability in coffee supplies means that a coffee taster's job is always changing.

Indonesia: Funk and Body

In place of Africa's hints of wine and fruit, Indonesia provides what Kevin Knox calls a "luscious herbal funk"—and also body, the hallmark of Indonesian coffees. The earthy notes result from the fact that most Indonesian coffee is dry-processed rather than washed, accentuating its already full body. The elusive taste that keeps Indonesia fans sampling bean after bean is not the fruity blackberry of Kenya but earthy wild mushroom.

Today three of the archipelago's islands produce coffee of world importance: Java, where the Dutch industry first and most famously took hold, Sulawesi and Sumatra. Sulawesi, often called by its old name, Celebes, is the favorite of buyers, for an elegance that sets it apart from other Indonesian coffees. Elegance in an unwashed coffee is pretty rare—and so are Sulawesi beans, because production is much lower on Sulawesi than on Java or Sumatra.

A name often attached automatically to Celebes is Kalossi, the coffee capital of a large growing region in the southwest part of the island called Toraja, where the native people, called Torajas, raise coffee trees on farms at various elevations. A very small amount of coffee from Toraja is washed, and it goes under the name of a Japanese company, Toarco, which owns a plantation and mill there. Although the Japanese have first call on these high-quality, washed beans, some come to the United States. Toraja beans have the famous Indonesian body and mushroomy flavors, and also an herbal finesse.

Sumatra beans are generally "semi-washed," meaning partly washed and partly dry-processed. The coffee is one of the most popular in the specialty trade, because of its massive body. Although less consistent and a bit cruder than Sulawesi, Sumatra is so powerful that it's hard to ruin. The two main growing regions on the island are Mandheling and Lintong. Some merchants used to make claims for the beans of one area over the other; because Mandheling was considered the classier region, merchants often put the name on the label. But the distinction is probably blurred at the shipping depot, as it is with the regions of Yemen, and of little importance to the consumer.

Sumatra also has one deluxe washed coffee, called Gayo Mountain for the area that in the 1980s was planted with trees of traditional varieties rather than modern, high-yielding ones. When it's good (some tasters say that in recent years quality has begun to dwindle, as the government has cut back its support for the project), Gayo Mountain offers an herbal clarity that appears only in washed coffees, with hints of a few sweet spices like clove and mace.

Java, synonymous with coffee, earns little respect from coffee people anymore. Most maintain that the planters of Java destroyed one of the world's great coffees by tearing down traditional trees starting in the 1970s and replacing them with higher-yielding plants. With this single, dramatic act, they deprived the world of one of its favorite coffees—one buyers relied on in order to brag about their true Mocha-Java blends. This was the final blow to an island that had already seen most of its old arabica trees replaced with robustas after an attack of disease, in 1876. During most of this century, only five government-owned plantations on Java even grew arabica beans; today the less said about the insipid beans on those estates, grown on high-yielding trees and machine-dried at high heat, the better.

Indonesia still offers many treasures, chief among them the beans of Sulawesi and Sumatra. A lesser-known treasure is aged coffee. Smallholders on both islands—most Indonesian farms are just an acre or two or three—keep bags of green coffee in their backyards as cash crops, to be sold when necessary. As a result of this hoarding, brokers can occasionally offer their customers aged coffees from either island, usually Sulawesi. Aged beans, always called "aged" on the store's bag or coffee menu, are expensive, but there's no way around the price. Because beans age better in the warm, damp climates in which they are grown, a merchant can't simply store them for two years in a warehouse (unless it is climate-controlled, which would be prohibitively expensive) and obtain the same flavor.

Aging emphasizes body and decreases acidity to near zero. Thus it is ideal for the already full-bodied Indonesian coffees, whose acids are rarely noteworthy to begin with; most of the herbal notes survive. Nothing is as soft as a good aged coffee. George Howell speaks of the range of flavors as being in dark, warm, golden tones, in contrast to the brighter colors of Kenyan and Costa Rican coffees. In aged Indonesias, the body is so thick as to be almost syrupy, regardless of the brewing method, but especially when brewed in a plunger pot. The plush, warm flavor can even make aged Sulawesi or Sumatra an alternative to an after-dinner liqueur.

New Guinea: Interesting Acidity

Coffee from Papua New Guinea, the eastern half of the island of New Guinea, above the northeastern tip of Australia, is usually categorized with Indonesia, because of its geographical proximity. But the fact that it is very carefully washed and that the rootstock is mostly from the exact varieties that made Jamaica Blue Mountain coffee legendary puts its style somewhere between Indonesia and Central America. The relatively recent start of the industry in Papua New Guinea and its rapid advancement give the coffee tremendous potential—some of which is already apparent in the cup.

At its best, New Guinea coffee has more pleasing and interesting acidity than any other Indonesia. This makes it more like a Central American coffee, except for its typically Indonesian heavy body and pronounced sweetness. New Guinea can be a helpful addition to an espresso blend, with the added bonus that it has heavier body than just about any washed arabica—a real advantage for espresso roasters like the premium Italian roaster, illycaffè, which insists on avoiding robusta in its espresso blends.

The finest New Guineas are both pleasing on their own and superb in a blend, complementing any acidic coffee and giving life to a dull one. Jerry Baldwin, of Peet's, told me that beans produced by the Sigri estate make the most complete coffee he knows—praise once reserved in the coffee trade for Jamaica Blue Mountain, which now seldom merits it. Each roaster announces with pride in its newsletters a shipment from one of these estates; fine Papua New Guinea beans also turn up on the menus of other specialty roasters.

India

India grows coffee, too, but so far it has not earned the admiration of specialty roasters, who dismiss it as poor man's Sumatra; the supply is more plentiful and lower-priced than the better Indonesian coffees. Still, the state of Mysore (now called Karnataka) has been producing arabicas since the mid-1600s, and quality beans are not unknown. Some shops will include Mysore for its name—as with Mocha, the old name is deemed more romantic—and to add some regional choice.

Also, the state of Malabar (now Kerala), from which Dutch colonizers first brought arabica trees to Java, is a consistent supplier of dry-processed, "monsooned" arabicas. These are stored in warehouses during the rainy season, a treatment that gives them many of the mellow, lightly spicy qualities people admire in aged Sulawesis and Sumatras; the supply from India is more consistent and cheaper.

Costa Rica and Guatemala: Legendary Completeness

A single tree—a fine arabica one at that—began the Western Hemisphere's mighty industry. It crossed the sea in 1723 under the care of an enterprising marine captain, Gabriel Mathieu de Clieu, who had heard how well coffee grew in Java and got the idea of bringing a tree back to Martinique, the Caribbean French colony where he was posted.

The story is so romantic that tale-spinners want to say he stole a tree by night and made off for his ship. But according to Gordon Wrigley's authoritative *Coffee,* it is more likely that Louis XV instructed de Clieu to try to grow the tree, which the unsuspecting Dutch had given him as a royal gift, on the island. The amazing fact remains that one tree—of an arabica species later named for Bourbon, the island in the Indian Ocean now called Réunion, then a French colony—gave life to hundreds of plantations spanning islands and continents.

Coffee blenders rely on Central and South American beans to give high notes to their blends. Crucial though Brazil is to the world's coffee supply—it produces around 30 percent of it—its bland, low-grown arabicas play a surprisingly minor role in the specialty trade. The even duller robusta beans that account for the coffee-growing industries of many other South American countries are also not very important. You won't find the names of Venezuela, Ecuador and Peru, for instance, on bins at specialty stores, although you might find, unbilled, their beans, which are cheap and useful in blends.

Instead, roasters focus on the beans of Central America, especially those of Costa Rica and Guatemala, which produce coffees of legendary completeness. It's hard to get a bad coffee from Costa Rica, which for the consistency of its processing is called the Switzerland of coffee-producing countries. Costa Rican beans are constantly in demand by German buyers, who for centuries have favored beautifully clean coffees, and by Americans who insist on the purest flavor. Coffee people keep track of tiny portions of the small country, favoring, say, the particularly bright coffees of Tres Rios or Dota, both part of Tarrazu, a large growing region near San José. All three names can appear on labels of Costa Rican coffees, but the most common is Tarrazu, since it encompasses so many beans.

Costa Rican coffee is rarely out of balance, neither too full-bodied relative to the acidity nor peculiarly acidic. It holds its own as it cools—quite a feat, since most coffees reveal their defects as they cool, when usually one or another characteristic comes to dominate. La Minita, the ultimate Costa Rican coffee, is clear as a bell, and even stone-cold, it stays sweet and beautifully pure. So immaculate are many Costa Rican beans, especially compared with the defect-ridden samples that arrive daily in buyers' cupping rooms, that the country draws a kind of reverse criticism: its coffee is too perfect.

Adventurers want a few funky notes, a few imperfections to put into dramatic relief the acidity or the deep body or the mocha-flavored overtones they love. For this they go to Guatemala, the country next door, whose coffees are loved as much as Costa Ricans are admired. The beans inspire adjectives like "smoky" and "chocolaty," providing a tantalizing counterpoint to what Howell calls "razor-fine acidity." The soil in the most noted growing region, Antigua (not to be confused with the Caribbean island of the same name, which does not grow coffee), is volcanic, like the soil of the Tarrazu region of Costa Rica. Antiguan coffees grow on volcanic hillsides an hour or so away from the capital, Guatemala City—hillsides that, coffee hands will tell you, are the most beautiful coffee terraces in the world.

The various regions of Guatemala have preserved their individuality better than those of Costa Rica, chiefly because Guatemala has more microclimates than Costa Rica, and climate strongly affects the character of beans. Too, Guatemalan farmers have not yet planted high-yielding hybrids, as many Costa Rican farmers have done. Instead, many Guatemalans have preserved their Bourbon trees, even going so far as to rip out newer varieties and replant traditional trees. (If only Java would do the same.)

A high region on the Gulf side of Guatemala, Cobán, grows beans in a far moister climate, which can result in fruitier flavors. Both "Antigua" and "Cobán" appear on menus as names of coffees, with no explanation that they both come from Guatemala. The geography can get even more specific, if an enthusiastic coffee buyer comes back to the shop from on-site tastings of Guatemalan beans. Kevin Knox, who searches for beans with character, once wrote in Allegro's newsletter of discovering in Guatemala the "sweet, sparkling and round coffees of the Fraijanes region" and "the powerful acidity and bitter-orange fruit of Huehuetenango."

In short, some would be happy to spend a lifetime drinking only Guatemalan coffee. They would often be disappointed by defects, because processing in Guatemala is not as careful as it is in Costa Rica. But when you hit a Guatemalan Antigua that is just right—with acidity, sweetness and enveloping body in perfect balance, and a veil of smokiness that gives the whole thing depth and mystery—you can be forgiven for never wanting to look further.

More from Central America

Mexico, bordering Guatemala, has recently tried to make forays into the specialty world, after years of being content to watch its beans go into mass-market blends. So far, choosy buyers aren't impressed. Acidity is lacking, and the beans are often low-grown and soft, making them unsuitable for anything darker than a medium roast. You'll frequently find Mexican coffees offered at specialty stores, because to buy Mexican beans is, as Jerry Baldwin says, "the neighborly thing to do." The name will frequently include the word *altura,* which simply means "high-grown" and suggests but does not guarantee good quality. The most flavorful beans come from Chiapas and Oaxaca, the growing regions nearest the Guatemalan border, where beans are washed. Although washing is the "fancy" way of preparing coffees, it removes the rough and earthy edges some people remember fondly from trips to Mexico: indeed, the great majority of Mexican beans are dry-processed.

Panama produces washed arabicas that most buyers put into blends. Mary Williams arranged to buy the entire production of one farm, La Florentina, for Starbucks, comparing it in acidity and body to a good but not great Costa Rican or Guatemalan coffee. Her peers, though, are only sometimes excited about anything they taste from Panama.

Two other Central American countries, Nicaragua and El Salvador, have in the past produced excellent arabicas from old Bourbon stocks. Many Bourbon trees were uprooted in Nicaragua, which in recent years has been renovating its coffee industry, privatizing it again after years of state control. Estate-grown coffees are just beginning to be sent to specialty roasters; if you find Nicaraguan beans marked with the name of the adjoining Matagalpa and Jinotega regions—or with the name of any estate—you'll likely taste coffee with the full body of a Caribbean bean and the powerful acidity of a Central America. Kevin Knox calls coffee Nicaragua's "industry of hope." El Salvador has been avoided by politically correct roasters, who object to the country's human-rights record. This is a valid objection, of course, but one that surprisingly doesn't seem to trouble the same roasters about Guatemala or other Central and South American countries where—as in Yemen, Uganda, Somalia, Indonesia and the Philippines, among other coffee-producing countries —the countries' attitudes toward human rights continue to be controversial.

South America: Image vs. Reality

The coffees of South America are much better known to the public than those of Central America, but are of relatively scant interest to specialty roasters. Colombia has been enormously successful in marketing itself as a producer of fine coffees by showing Juan Valdez and his mule trudging up mountainsides, and the country's washed arabicas are consistently well processed. But specialty merchants must look long and hard to find anything they'd think of selling to be brewed alone. At best, Colombias are clean and neutral—good for blends in which they will give moderate acidity and body, and often a sweetness that some describe as caramel-like. As part of its emphasis on efficiency in the 1970s, Colombia embarked on a very ambitious replanting program, replacing old trees with Variedad Colombia, a new variety named for the country. Tasters agree that this variety, which is now being planted in other efficiency-minded countries, produces a blander bean than older varieties. Like Java, once Colombia ripped out old trees, it faded from the map of devoted coffee lovers.

One area, however, Nariño, has maintained older varieties and has recently taken special care in processing its beans. Colombia Nariño Supremo, to which Starbucks has exclusive rights, can be a superb coffee, offering the clear, well-defined acidity notable in most Costa Ricans, and fruity notes too. George Howell says that this coffee and a similar one marketed as Reserva del Patron must be drunk young, like Beaujolais wine, because they quickly lose their acidity.

Brazilian beans can ensure crema, the prized foam atop a cup of espresso, without the presence of robusta, the usual route to it. And they can also give a peculiar, hard flavor of iodine, associated with the coffees shipped from Rio de Janeiro. (As with other countries, Brazilian coffee names derive from ports, chiefly Rio, Santos and Bahia.) Buyers usually consider this a terrible defect, but certain places have acquired a taste for it—chiefly New Orleans, where the sour, peppery taste of chicory, a cheap filler, has come to be appreciated, and Turkey, which at the end of the nineteenth century began buying Rios because coffees from the Arabian Peninsula and Africa became too expensive.

A few pioneers have been working since the mid-1980s to change the course of Brazilian coffee. Now that the longstanding champion in bean production is being challenged by sudden newcomer Vietnam, the rest of Brazil's growers are taking note. Luis Norberto Pascoal, a Brazilian businessman and coffee grower, and Ernesto Illy, the indefatigable innovator and head of illycaffè, have separately and together perfected a means of processing arabica coffee cherries which allows the beans to absorb a bit of the *miel*, or mucilage, as they dry. The "pulp natural" process, which allows for carefully controlled sun drying, gives beans greater body without heightened acidity—big advantages to quality-minded roasters like Illy, who seek heavy-bodied espresso without resorting to low-flavor robusta beans. They are also designing new picking and sorting equipment to ensure that only ripe cherries get picked, something that was impossible with indiscriminate mechanical pickers. Coffees long dismissed as fit only for blending might one day take their place among their prized South American relatives.

The Caribbean: Misleading Mythology

The Caribbean, landing point of the first beans in the Western Hemisphere, has diminished in importance as a coffee-growing region. The most famous Caribbean coffee is that of Jamaica, which, unlike most other islands, has mountains high enough to produce superb beans—the Blue Mountains, home sweet home to any coffee snob who doesn't know much.

Here's a piece of advice: don't spend a fortune on a bean labeled Jamaica Blue Mountain to find that rarer-than-rare balance of acidity and body, fruit and spice that so enchanted generations of coffee drinkers. You can better spend your time and money looking for a great Guatemala or Costa Rica.

The myth of Jamaica Blue Mountain lives on because the coffee continues to be scarce and expensive. Naturally, anything that costs so much—up to $40 a pound at retail, making it the caviar of coffees—must be the best there is. A sample of Blue Mountain coffee from the best estate might legitimately recall the legend. But you'll have to spend a small fortune to get a taste. The important thing to remember is that you're not missing anything you can't get from other countries at a fraction of the price.

Vague, misleading words like "mountain blend" mean that you won't find a Blue Mountain bean in the bag. Jamaica High Mountain is a common, boring coffee, but the name, an official government-designated grade, is similar enough to Blue Mountain to fool plenty of consumers. If, by some accident, true Blue Mountain does play a part in any of the many blends that claim to feature it, professional tasters would be hard-pressed to confirm the fact—even genuine Blue Mountain often tastes like just another Central. Donald N. Schoenholt, a coffee authority and historian and scion of Gillies Coffee Company, in Brooklyn, which calls itself America's Oldest Coffee Merchant, defends genuine Blue Mountain as "exquisite when it is good." The price, he points out, is so high because it is "the rarest of the arabica beans with the potential for greatness." (A sure way to know you're evaluating the real thing is to order from J. Martinez, originally coffee growers in Jamaica and now in Atlanta; see Sources, page 252.)

Few of the other islands produce noteworthy coffees. Those from the Dominican Republic, usually called Santo Domingo, can be perfectly respectable. Some recent arrivals offer viscous body when brewed, like the majority of Caribbean beans, and relatively high acidity. Knox says that good Caribbean coffees are syrupy and raisin-sweet, with the mellowness of Spanish brandies. They are at their best in a medium-dark roast, which accentuates their sweetness. Of the Caribbean beans that arrive in the United States, Puerto Rico's are notable, as the island has begun a large effort to revitalize its coffee industry (at U.S. labor prices, the effort is expensive). So far, the beans from two farms, sold under the name Yauco Selecto, are the most promising.

These islands have traditionally made the best of their low-grown, low-acid beans by roasting them dark. Visitors come back from Cuba and Puerto Rico raving about subtle, sweet, dark coffee. Indeed, these coffees taste like no one else's, happily lacking the harsh, charred overtones so often notable in dark roasts. Their softness shows best in a plunger pot or a stovetop or steam-powered espresso machine.

Hawaii

The Caribbean is generally grouped with the other coffee legend, Hawaii, the source of the only coffee grown in the United States. Kona coffee, which is cultivated on the volcanic slopes of Mauna Loa, is scarce and expensive because of Hawaii's astronomical labor costs, and the real stuff rarely plays any significant part in a blend that uses the name. Like Jamaica Blue Mountain, even the genuine article varies in the interest it merits. Bean quality is uniformly high, because processing is careful everywhere. As for flavor, the acidity in most Kona coffees that outsiders taste is flat and the body light.

Any Kona with real flavor is virtually impossible to find outside Hawaii. Unlike any other coffee-growing area, Hawaii saves the best for itself, because it can make the most profit by selling locally and to tourists.

Inspired Blends

Few coffees have everything. Only a very few coffees from Kenya, Costa Rica and Guatemala have the snap of sharp acidity, the mellowness of full body and spice and fruit notes too—the works. It's nearly impossible to find any other complete single-origin coffee. For that reason, even after tasting around the world at your local specialty-coffee store, chances are you'll wind up with a blend, either of the store's or your own devising.

The world of fine coffee is divided into people who think in terms of blends and people who persist in looking for perfection in a single coffee. It's possible to combine both loves, but inspired blends usually come from people such as Jerry Baldwin, who, upon tasting something they really like, say, "You know what would be good with that?" Baldwin likes to reminisce about the time he found a good Jamaica Blue Mountain. He rushed to the blending room, assembling one-third Blue Mountain, one-third Mocha Sanani and one-third Costa Rican. "It was pretty damn tasty," he says.

His spur-of-the-moment creation shows the instincts of an experienced blender. (It also shows a sky's-the-limit imagination.) A good Blue Mountain, a washed coffee, has medium body and fairly bright but not electric acidity. The Mocha Sanani, an unwashed bean, would add a full body that no washed coffee could ever provide, and wild notes that such a carefully processed bean could never supply. The Costa Rican would emphasize acidity.

Someone blending for flavor, then, will think about each bean and what will fill in the missing notes, whether they be spice, wine, fruit, rich body or flowery delicacy. Too much of one trait—the heavy body of a Sumatra, say—can wipe out a different trait, like the floral notes of an Ethiopian Yergacheffe. Two beans with similar and special traits—the berry flavors of Kenya and Ethiopian Harrar, for instance—might cancel each other out. This leads to a general rule that similar flavor ranges don't go together.

Most merchants don't work with such stellar components. The goal is to keep down costs by devising a pleasing blend that can change according to what's available and what's cheap. Blenders who can do this on a grand scale earn the grandest salaries.

Few home brewers want to bother with the fine points of blending: that's what a roaster is for. Still, if you try to make your own Mocha-Java, you'll give yourself an introductory course in blending and be a more discerning judge of other people's blends. The standard formula is half Java and half Mocha, although for the past decades, the high price and scarcity of Mocha has pushed down its percentage to one-third Mocha against two-thirds Java. The idea is that the full body of Java will be the sturdy pedestal upon which the gamy, earthy notes of the Mocha rest.

Since good Java, too, is hard to come by, the logical substitution is a Sulawesi or New Guinea or Sumatra. And in place of the scarce Mocha, you can try an Ethiopian Harrar. Or you can add an Ethiopian Sidamo or Yerga-cheffe—washed coffees with far greater finesse. It's always interesting to play the purity, medium body and high acidity of a washed coffee like a Central American against the wildness of an unwashed coffee, like an Ethiopian or a Yemen. If you find a New Guinea Sigri estate, you can try adding the acidity of a Kenya or Costa Rican, or the earthy funk of a Sumatra, or the wininess of a true Mocha.

Lay in a supply of two or three coffees you enjoy, and vary the proportion of scoops in each morning's pot of coffee, taking notes on the day's experiment. You'll soon find a whole that is far greater than the sum of its parts.

8

Caffeine and Decaf

P RACTICALLY EVERYONE RELIES ON CAFFEINE to keep going: a 1984 study called it the most widely used behaviorally active drug in the world. Fully 80 percent of American adults consume enough to make a difference in the way they feel and act every day. It is estimated that the average U.S. adult ingests about 200 milligrams of caffeine daily—the amount in two cups of coffee.

A drug that almost everyone needs has naturally attracted an enormous amount of attention from researchers. What harm does it do? Can it increase someone's risk of contracting a life-threatening disease, or worsen the effects of one? Does the fact that so many people can't get through the day without consuming caffeine mean that it should be considered addictive, or that it should even be called a drug of abuse?

So far, virtually every attempt to link caffeine to a life-threatening disease has either come to nothing or had such ambiguous results that researchers have presumed the link to be absent. No organization devoted to a specific disease—no major medical organization, in fact—has cautioned against consuming caffeine.

This does not mean that everyone in the medical profession considers caffeine to be innocent. Doctors and nurses routinely counsel some patients to watch their caffeine intake or eliminate it altogether. They base their concerns on personal experience, stories their patients tell them, or on confusing studies they've read, and decide to err on the conservative side. And for pregnant women, there are reasons to be wary of caffeine and to consider eliminating it.

An awareness of the hazards of caffeine to mental well-being is beginning to emerge among psychiatrists and general practitioners. What people have for years called "caffeine jitters"—the feeling of wanting to jump out of your skin if you consume too much caffeine—now has an official diagnosis, Caffeine Intoxication, listed in the most recent edition of the psychiatrist's handbook, the *Diagnostic and Statistical Manual of Mental Disorders*. Its most common symptoms include anxiety, insomnia, gastrointestinal disturbances and tremors.

Some researchers argue that the manual should also define Caffeine Withdrawal, the side effect most likely to affect anyone who tries to give up caffeine. Relatively few people experience Caffeine Intoxication, although its exact prevalence in the general population has never been studied. But almost anyone who has given up caffeine knows the fierce headache that can last a day or two, along with drowsiness and a general lack of interest in life.

Should you aim to renounce caffeine and switch to decaf? Definitive advice is impossible to come by. Scientists don't know how and why caffeine has the effects it does. Their knowledge of the way it acts on the brain and the body, though, is more complete than their knowledge of any health risks it might pose. Understanding how caffeine makes you feel after you drink it—and, especially, after you stop drinking it—will probably give you a better idea of whether to keep consuming it than will tackling the hundreds of contradictory and inconclusive studies on possible links between caffeine and major diseases.

It's important to keep two things in mind about the effects of drinking coffee. First, caffeine is only its most active and studied component. The many acids in coffee—especially chlorogenic acid, which appears in higher quantity in inexpensive robusta beans than it does in higher-quality arabica beans—speed up the digestive process and can cause gastric irritation. These components remain in decaffeinated coffee. Most studies don't distinguish between caffeinated and decaffeinated coffee, a potentially important flaw.

The other thing to remember is that in the absence of definitive health warnings against coffee, you'll have to make up your own mind about how much to drink in a day. However contradictory they may be, the hundreds of studies continually underline the fact that reactions to caffeine vary tremendously by individual. If you think that drinking coffee anytime after noon will keep you awake, you're probably right. If you brag that you'll enjoy the sleep of the innocent following a double after-dinner espresso, you're probably also right—and lucky. Everyone knows somebody infuriating like the woman I once met in Brazil who told me, "If I'm sleepy, I take a coffee. If I wake up at night and want to get back to sleep, I take a coffee."

The Power of Caffeine

The prevailing theory of why caffeine increases alertness took shape only in the early 1970s. The theory holds that caffeine interferes with the depressant effects of adenosine, which is one of the chemicals that the body makes to control neural activity. Adenosine triggers a series of slowing effects: it depresses mood and alertness, lowers the need to urinate and slows gastric secretion and respiration. After it is released by nerve endings in the brain, adenosine must reach receptors on the surface of certain brain cells in order to work. Caffeine, the theory has it, acts as an adenosine impostor. Molecules of caffeine counterfeit molecules of adenosine, locking into the adenosine receptors on brain cells. They fool the body into thinking that adenosine is circulating, but they produce no depressive effect of their own.

Caffeine speeds you up, then, by not slowing you down. Its effects are the opposite of adenosine's: caffeine makes you feel brighter and more alert, increases gastric secretion, makes you urinate more and stimulates respiration.

Proponents of caffeine speak of its ability to increase vigilance and heighten the ability to perform various tasks. Its effects are most pronounced, however, when compared with performance levels that are low because of fatigue, boredom or caffeine abstinence.

Despite the generations of writers who have thought that coffee helped them think more clearly, caffeine seems only to increase intellectual speed, not intellectual power. Subjects in experiments do things like read and fill out crossword puzzles faster—but not, unfortunately, more accurately.

Caffeine quickens reaction time and can enhance both hand-eye coordination and the capacity of muscles to work. This boost to overall endurance has led to its use by cyclists and runners. But caffeine also has a diuretic effect, increasing frequency of urination. Caffeinated drinks are thus dehydrating, good for neither athletes nor flyers (dehydration is one of the worst problems of air travel and a prime cause of jet lag).

Caffeine speeds up the metabolism and makes you burn calories faster, although not so much faster that it will help you lose weight. Its inclusion in over-the-counter diet pills in place of prescription-only amphetamines seems to be largely ineffective. Amphetamines, which diminish appetite, work differently from the way caffeine does on the brain.

This general quickening does not mean that coffee can sober you up— either black or with milk. Your motor functions will be just as impaired by alcohol as they were minutes before you downed that cup of coffee. Even if you feel more awake, you're just as dangerous a driver. Similarly, caffeine does not counteract the effects of phenobarbital and other barbiturates. It does, however, help reverse the impairment of cognitive activity caused by benzodiazepines, the compounds that are the basis of Valium and many other tranquilizers. Some researchers speculate that a similar restorative effect on cognitive activity might take place in the interaction between caffeine and alcohol, but no one yet knows. Remember, though, that the question to be studied is whether caffeine can help you *think* more clearly after you have drunk alcohol—not whether it will improve your reflexes. No one imagines that coffee can make you a safer driver after you've been drinking.

Besides being a self-prescribed antidepressant and alertness drug, caffeine has been shown to be useful to people with asthma, since it works as a bronchodilator, meaning that it widens the air passages in the lungs and eases breathing. It might even be something of an aphrodisiac, if the results of a University of Michigan study can be generally applied: the study showed that older subjects were more likely to be sexually active if they were coffee drinkers than if they were not.

Calculating Your Consumption

How much caffeine does it take to produce any of these effects? The answer, as studies progress, seems to be an ever smaller amount. Until recently, the behaviorally active dose was thought to be 85 milligrams of caffeine, roughly the amount in a small (5-ounce) cup of filter-brewed coffee. But new studies show that far smaller amounts—as little as 25 milligrams—can produce notable effects on alertness.

Measuring how much caffeine you consume is usually a matter of rough estimation. It's easier to say for sure how much caffeine you get from a soft drink or headache pill than from a cup of coffee, because the amount of caffeine varies by brewing method and by the kind of bean. Robusta beans contain twice as much caffeine as arabica beans.

An authoritative review chapter on caffeine from *Psychiatry,* a textbook written to accompany the *Diagnostic and Statistical Manual,* says that a 6-ounce cup of brewed coffee contains 100 milligrams of caffeine; again, variation is great. A single shot (1½ to 2 ounces) of espresso contains 80 to 100 milligrams—about the same as in the 6-ounce cup of brewed coffee.

It's wrong, then, to think that a serving of espresso has more caffeine than a serving of coffee. The reason the amounts are nearly identical is that about the same amount of beans by weight are used to brew a 6-ounce cup of filtered coffee as a single espresso. Hot water is such an efficient solvent for caffeine that simply passing hot water through ground coffee gets nearly all the caffeine out, whatever the brewing method. If you have a cappuccino or a caffè latte at an espresso bar, the milk-diluted drink will likely contain far less caffeine than the same volume of black filter-brewed coffee.

Not only do the estimates of how much caffeine coffee contains vary, but the 5- to 6-ounce serving size they assume is utterly foreign to most Americans. A standard take-out cup of filter-brewed coffee is 12 ounces, and a "large" cup is often a whopping 20 ounces. Similarly, most American espresso bars serve a "plain" espresso as a double shot and use a double shot in cappuccinos and caffè lattes. (In Italy, an espresso is a single shot, whatever the drink.)

Brewed tea contains less caffeine than brewed coffee, even though tea leaves by weight can have double the amount of caffeine as coffee beans. The reason is that less tea is used in brewing. A 6-ounce cup of tea typically contains 40 milligrams of caffeine, although, as with coffee, there is variation by type. Black tea, the familiar kind, has been fermented and oxidized and contains more caffeine by weight than oolong tea, which is only partially fermented, or green tea.

Most cola drinks contain between 38 and 45 milligrams of caffeine per 12-ounce serving, as compared with about 200 milligrams in the same amount of coffee. Some sodas have more: Mountain Dew, for instance, has 54 milligrams in 12 ounces. Manufacturers claim that they add caffeine for the taste and not to woo coffee drinkers. But in fact, starting in the early 1960s, coffee consumption declined while soft-drink consumption skyrocketed. Caffeine *does* have a taste—it's bitter. That may sound unpleasant, but try tasting a caffeinated cola against its caffeine-free version, looking for the balance of bitter to sweet.

Over-the-counter pain relievers, too, are a considerable source of caffeine: a single dose of two pills can contain 50 to 130 milligrams. The reason so many of these remedies include caffeine is that it is thought to speed and magnify the effects of pain relief, although no study has definitively shown that it does.

Many studies suggest that people regulate the amount of caffeine they consume, consciously or unconsciously, in order to get what they seek without feeling jittery or drowsy. Several studies show a curious sidelight, though: some people react to a caffeinated drink or pill based on what they are told they have consumed rather than what they actually have consumed. This would comfort the scores of restaurant managers who think that customers already make too big a deal out of whether or not they get decaf after dinner.

Sleepless Nights

Of course, the effects of caffeine are not imaginary, especially not on sleep. If they were, millions of people wouldn't be so dependent on caffeine to get them going and wouldn't worry about drinking it at night. Most studies confirm what everyone knows—coffee not only makes you alert, it keeps you awake. It also often decreases total sleep time and increases the number of times you waken in the night, depending on how much you drink and especially on how sensitive you are to it.

Although caffeine does interfere with some sleep stages and lessens the quality of sleep, it has been shown in many studies not to decrease rapid-eye-movement sleep, the restorative kind, the way as alcohol and barbiturates do. Sleep disturbance from caffeine seems to be more severe in older people, which is one reason that consumption of decaffeinated coffee increases with age; in general, people seem to become more sensitive to caffeine as they grow older.

Individual sensitivity extends to how long it takes someone to metabolize caffeine, so there's no general cutoff time for when to drink the last cup of coffee if you want to sleep well. The body absorbs caffeine almost completely, and fast—it appears in all tissue fluids about five minutes after it is ingested and reaches its highest levels after thirty to sixty minutes. But the body gets rid of caffeine relatively slowly, and the time it takes the liver to break down and the kidney to expel caffeine in urine varies from person to person. The average half-life of caffeine in the body, meaning the time it takes the body to eliminate half the caffeine ingested, is four to six hours. Given a standard half-life of five hours, active levels of caffeine will remain in the body for more than ten to fifteen hours, depending on a person's sensitivity. Studies of the disruptions to sleep have found that its effects can last even longer—twenty-four hours or more.

Heavy smokers clear caffeine twice as fast, which might be one of many reasons that smoking and heavy coffee drinking have been strongly associated. Smokers, that is, may need to consume more caffeine to feel the same effects as nonsmokers. The longtime correlation between caffeine and smoking has been one of the many rocks in the reef of caffeine studies. Time and again, harmful effects claimed for caffeine have turned out to be the masked effects of smoking.

Withdrawal Pangs

It's striking that after decades of inconclusive research into the possible long-term threats of caffeine to life span, researchers took so long to examine coffee drinking's most obvious and debilitating side effect: once you become habituated to caffeine, a matter of days, you can feel rotten when you stop consuming it. Recent studies show withdrawal to be both worse and more common than most doctors know. Light drinkers aren't exempt: studies reveal that withdrawal takes place even after cessation of very small amounts of caffeine—100 milligrams, the amount in a 6-ounce cup of coffee.

By far the commonest symptom of withdrawal is a headache, which can start just a few hours after caffeine is stopped but is usually worst after between twenty and forty-eight hours. In a study featured in a 1992 issue of the *New England Journal of Medicine,* conducted by a group including Roland R. Griffiths, a longtime caffeine researcher at Johns Hopkins University School of Medicine, over half the subjects reported moderate or severe headaches when they were given placebo tablets rather than tablets containing caffeine.

Often the headache lasts one to two days. The adenosine-receptor theory says that long-term caffeine consumption creates more receptor sites for adenosine, as the body starts sensing the relative lack of the depressant and tunes up its sensitivity. When caffeine stops, so does impostor adenosine, and the body becomes hypersensitive to real adenosine. The theory has it that cerebral blood flow increases with the increased activity of real adenosine. Headache and loginess result. With time, the headache goes away, because the body compensates by cutting back the number of adenosine receptors to the pre-caffeine level. It takes two days to a week to get over caffeine withdrawal completely, according to most estimates.

Headache can be just one part of the miseries of withdrawal. According to a 1995 psychopharmacology textbook by Griffiths, other symptoms, in rough order of frequency after headache, include drowsiness; difficulty working and concentrating; decreased self-confidence and increased irritability; decreased sociability and friendliness; flulike feelings, including muscle aches, hot or cold spells, heavy feelings in arms or legs; nausea; and blurred vision. Subjects deprived of caffeine in the Griffiths study reported similar complaints: "I couldn't concentrate . . . I'm basically not a low person; [I was] mildly sad and depressed." Another subject felt "sad, uncertain about the future . . . glum." Or, "I felt like I had the flu, a severe headache, extreme fatigue." People who stop caffeine feel lousy.

The subjects in the study fell into the low to moderate range of caffeine consumption, whereas previous studies of dependence and withdrawal had been focused on heavy coffee drinkers. The results suggested that caffeine withdrawal is far more common than most clinicians realized, and Griffiths and his fellow researchers recommended that doctors keep caffeine withdrawal in mind when patients report headache, fatigue or mood disturbances. The study also noted that doctors should realize that complaints of headaches before and after surgical procedures may simply reflect the required abstinence from all beverages beforehand. The authors suggested that doctors should consider recommending caffeine supplements to spare patients headaches, since caffeine is known to have a constricting effect on dilated blood vessels in the brain. If a doctor wants to tell patients to cut out all caffeine, the study also said, the reduction should be gradual and not abrupt.

Is It Addictive?

Even if withdrawal symptoms usually end within a week, many people find it hard to give up caffeine for good, despite a doctor's advice. So is caffeine addictive? The matter is thorny, because different people have different definitions of addiction. The withdrawal syndrome that caffeine produces means that it can be said to induce physical dependence. That isn't the same as saying that someone is "clinically dependent" on a drug, which means the person uses it pathologically. Although many people use the terms "drug of dependence" and "drug of abuse" interchangeably, an abused drug is usually defined as one whose use harms both the user and society.

According to an overview chapter on caffeine and the central nervous system by Kenneth Hirsh in *Methylxanthine Beverages and Foods*, the central nervous system and many other organ systems quickly develop tolerance to the effects of caffeine. When someone "tolerates" a drug, he or she needs more of it to produce the same effect. Hirsh wrote, "All definitions of addiction . . . eventually boil down to compulsion with and for a drug. [Caffeine] simply [does] not support such behavior."

Although Griffiths agrees that caffeine does not strictly qualify as an addictive drug, he points to its "reinforcing" effect—its tendency to create dependence. In a later study of people who identified themselves as having trouble giving up caffeine, Griffiths suggested that caffeine dependence be added to the American Psychiatric Association diagnostics manual; it will appear after 2010.

Unlike many addictive drugs, caffeine does not stimulate an appetite for ever-higher doses. People seem to take it repeatedly when the doses are small, but taper off as the doses go beyond 50 to 100 milligrams at a time—a mere cup of filter-brewed coffee or single shot of espresso. After receiving a very large dose, such as 400 to 600 milligrams, people often avoid caffeine altogether for a while. Most find the dose they like and consume neither less nor more of it.

A Clean Report Card

Frank evaluation of the hazards of caffeine and coffee is as thorny as assessing their addictive qualities. Besides the headache and flulike symptoms of caffeine withdrawal, about the only health connection that can be made with certainty is that coffee can cause stomach pain and heartburn. Researchers suspect that caffeine leads to the secretion of gastric acids by blocking the effects of adenosine, which slows down gastrointestinal activity. Whether caffeine alone or another substance in coffee produces the gastric secretion remains a question; it seems likely that other components are also at work, because decaffeinated coffee can cause the same effects. One study found that coffee and decaffeinated coffee were each twice as strong in producing gastrointestinal effects as caffeine alone. The role of coffee and caffeine in ulcers has been little studied: they are not thought to cause ulcers, though both are known to make them worse. Coffee's laxative effect, which some people depend on, has been found in both caffeinated and decaffeinated coffee. Again, your own experience is the best guide.

There is a vast literature on the effects of caffeine on the body and its possible dangers, and little of it agrees with the rest. Most major health risks have been ruled out, however. Along with reassurances that emerge from "meta-surveys"—articles that tabulate and analyze the findings of hundreds of studies—come clean report cards from groups like the National Academy of Sciences National Research Council and the U.S. Surgeon General's office. All say that no association has been established between moderate caffeine consumption and an increased risk to health.

Easing Heartfelt Concerns

Still, researchers keep looking into certain diseases—most often, heart disease. Caffeine has been associated with irregular heartbeats when consumed at extremely high levels; it raises blood pressure temporarily, and it has been suspected of raising cholesterol levels. Heart disease is still America's leading fatal disease, and public alarm about cholesterol has fueled research into links with caffeine and coffee.

Study after study finds no meaningful link. Why devote limited resources to keep looking for one? I asked this of Walter Willett, one of the country's leading nutritional epidemiologists, as he was about to submit for publication data from the Nurses' Health Study, which has been tracking the dietary habits of more than 85,000 female nurses since 1980. The results cleared caffeine of increasing the risk of heart disease—an important echo of the 1990 Harvard Health Professionals' Study of 45,000 men, which showed no association between coffee consumption and heart disease or stroke.

Willett, who is the chair of the Department of Nutrition at the Harvard School of Public Health, helped direct the men's study. "The main message here," he said, "is that for people drinking up to six cups a day, there is no strong reason to give up coffee and, particularly, no strong reason to switch to decaf."

Even if that statement seemed to close the case, Willett pursued the matter, he told me, because that study was only of men, and the women's study was already under way. Also, he said, at the time of the publication of the men's study, there was concern that decaffeinated coffee might somehow be a risk factor for heart disease. The Nurses' Health Study definitively showed that decaffeinated coffee plays no role in increased risk of heart disease.

For the past twenty years, other large and well-conducted studies have reiterated that there is no connection between caffeine, coffee and heart disease. A 1992 meta-analysis of large studies conducted between 1966 and 1991 and involving 103,000 people in six countries, published by Martin

Myers and Antoni Basinki at the Sunnybrook Medical Center, in Toronto, strongly concluded that coffee consumption does not contribute to heart disease. This finding was corroborated a year later by results from the Scottish Heart Health Study. As early as 1974, a twelve-year study as part of the Framingham Heart Study concluded that there was no association between coffee and heart attacks, coronary heart disease, angina pectoris or sudden death.

The search for another cholesterol-raising villain goes on, though. A 1989 study reported that subjects who drank decaffeinated coffee experienced a rise in serum cholesterol. The medical community dismissed the study as incomplete and based on too few people, and larger subsequent studies like those at Harvard failed to support the link.

One reason researchers have doggedly pursued the connection is that a 1991 study, published in the Netherlands, found that in Scandinavian countries, coffee significantly raised cholesterol. The results worried people all over the world until the mystery was solved in 1994: the culprit was two lipids that appear in coffee, called cafestol and kahweol, but that appear in quantity only in boiled coffee—the kind popular in northern Europe. Filters remove more than 80 percent of the substances, so concern in most other countries is needless. Puzzles are rarely solved so neatly.

Still, doubt remains in the public mind, and research goes on. "You know how every artist at some point has to paint a bowl of fruit?" Walt Willett asked me. "Well, caffeine and heart disease is a nutritional researcher's bowl of fruit."

The Cancer Scare

Similarly, the hunt for a link between caffeine and coffee and any kind of cancer—bladder, rectal, colon, urinary tract and kidney in particular—has been intensive. In 1992, the chief of environmental epidemiology at the National Cancer Institute, Robert N. Hoover, expressed the common opinion among researchers: "There is no good evidence of a causal relationship between coffee and any type of cancer."

The first and most famous health scare about coffee associated it with pancreatic cancer, in 1981. This turned out to be another case of missing links. "Confounding factors," as they are known, such as preexisting gastrointestinal conditions, cigarette smoking and a sedentary existence, were not taken into account. Five years later, the authors took back their original findings—a rare event in the competitive world of epidemiology—but their update received little attention. Many subsequent studies have also ruled out any increased risk of pancreatic cancer from caffeine consumption; a 1991 study in Montreal found that coffee drinkers had a *lower* risk of pancreatic cancer than nondrinkers. But the initial public alarm never completely faded.

Researchers have largely given up on caffeine and breast cancer, as study after study dismisses it as a subject for concern. In 1993, for instance, the Iowa Women's Health Study, which followed 34,388 older women for four years, found no association between caffeine consumption and the risk of breast cancer. A meta-analysis of studies from forty-four countries, published in 1988 by researchers at the University of Rochester, did not turn up a link between breast cancer and caffeine from coffee or tea.

A connection between drinking coffee and benign breast disease, or fibrocystic disease, remains controversial among the public and among some doctors and nurses, even if the research community has dismissed it. Concern was raised initially by a 1979 study of forty-seven women, but later studies did not uphold its results, especially a large study conducted by researchers from the National Cancer Institute, reported in 1986. Both the National Cancer Institute and the American Medical Association's Council on Scientific Affairs have said that there is no association between caffeine intake and fibrocystic breast disease.

Prudence During Pregnancy

If coffee's role in breast cancer and fibrocystic disease has been discounted, its effects on fertility and spontaneous abortions have not. Caffeine crosses the placenta and enters the fetus, and pregnant women clear caffeine from their bodies slowly—twice as slowly during the second trimester, and three times as slowly during the third trimester, as when they are not pregnant. In 1980, the Food and Drug Administration advised pregnant women and those who might become pregnant to reduce or eliminate caffeine, citing evidence from animal studies that it caused birth defects, fetal death and low birth weights. The advice was based largely on an FDA experiment in which pregnant rats, force-fed through a stomach tube with the equivalents of fifty-six and eighty-seven cups of strong coffee at one time, gave birth to offspring with missing toes or parts of toes. However, a later study giving rats the same exaggerated doses, this time in drinking water and at a modified rate over a day, showed none of the birth defects.

The FDA did not alter its advice, even though a 1982 study of 2,030 women found no relation between caffeine consumption during pregnancy and six specific birth defects, and a 1988 review of thirteen studies on humans conducted between 1981 and 1988, compiled by researchers at Boston's Children's Hospital, showed "no evidence . . . that caffeine consumption at moderate levels by pregnant women has any discernible adverse effect on their fetuses."

In 1993, the issue again became charged, as the *Journal of the American Medical Association* published two large studies with conflicting advice. The first, conducted by researchers at the National Institute of Child Health and reported in February, reassured pregnant women that if they consumed under 300 milligrams of caffeine a day, which is to say less than two or three cups of coffee, they stood no greater risk of miscarrying or bearing low-birth-weight babies than women who abstained.

Then, the following December, a study from McGill University, in Montreal, which contrasted a group of women whose pregnancies ended in miscarriage with a group of pregnant women who carried to term, found that the risk of miscarriage jumped more than 20 percent for each 100 milligrams of caffeine a pregnant woman ingested daily. An accompanying editorial by a researcher at the University of California at Berkeley offered a few explanations of how the two large studies could come to such different conclusions. The Canadian study did not control for nausea during pregnancy, which frequently provokes women to give up coffee; women with troubled pregnancies generally experience less nausea and therefore continue to drink their normal amount of coffee. Perhaps the measurements of caffeine, too, were inexact, as they are in many studies.

Many such quarrels with the methodology and conclusions of the Canadian study were raised in the months following the study's publication. But unless the results of the Canadian study are conclusively overturned, pregnant women are likely to adhere to the editorial's conclusion: daily consumption of over 300 milligrams of coffee might be risky during pregnancy, and lower levels cannot be guaranteed safe either. Since the Canadian study found that even in the months before pregnancy, caffeine could increase the risk of miscarriage, and other studies had suggested that high caffeine consumption could retard conception, the editorial ended by saying that women trying to conceive and pregnant women would be prudent to follow the 1980 FDA guidelines and keep caffeine consumption to a minimum.

Lingering Questions

Still under investigation is the relationship between caffeine consumption and osteoporosis, the disease that affects many older women, causing bones to become porous and brittle. Caffeine is known to increase calcium excretion. But several studies, including a 1992 Mayo Clinic study and another in the same year examining a population of 619 men and women in their seventies, found that caffeine consumption did not elevate the risk of osteoporosis.

A 1994 study at the University of California at San Diego of nearly a thousand older women found that although a woman's consumption of caffeine definitely corresponded to a decrease in bone density in the hips and spine, there was no such correspondence in women who drank at least a glass of milk a day during their adult life.

While further studies remain to be completed, then, the current advice is for women not to give up caffeine but to be sure to eat as many calcium-rich foods, such as skim milk, yogurt and cheese, as possible. This is especially important in early adulthood, when women are still building bone mass.

The Switch to Decaf

Whether or not caffeine is hazardous or truly addictive, becoming habituated to it and suffering coffee nerves or caffeine withdrawal is no fun, and many people have chosen to drink decaffeinated coffee instead. In 1962, the peak year for American coffee consumption, decaffeinated coffee made up only 3 percent of coffee sales; today it accounts for 20 percent.

It's a shame that most decaffeinated coffee is so terrible, because it doesn't have to be. Traditionally, inferior robusta beans have been chosen for decaffeination, because they yield more caffeine, which is sold at a high price to soft-drink and patent-medicine companies. Also, robusta beans have more body when they are brewed, and so after they are decaffeinated they will seem less like brown water. Now many kinds of the superior arabica beans are being decaffeinated in ways that conserve both flavor and body. But the public suffers from an unwarranted fear of the process that leaves in the most taste—chemical decaffeination—and prefers instead to buy water-processed decaf.

Decaffeination has been practiced since the turn of the century. Every process, whether chemical- or water-based, starts with steaming the green (unroasted) beans to loosen the bonds of caffeine. In the chemical process, a solvent circulates through the beans, coming into direct contact with them and carrying the caffeine with it. The drained solvent is then mixed with water, and the caffeine is extracted to be sold. The beans are again steamed, to remove any residual solvent, and dried. Like all green beans, they are then sold to be roasted.

In the water process, no solvent touches the beans. After the beans are steamed, they are soaked in water in big vats, which removes the caffeine—along with all the soluble solids in the beans. The solution is drained off to a separate tank, where the caffeine is extracted from it. While the caffeine is being removed, the beans sit devoid of everything that gives them flavor. At the end, the beans are resoaked with the decaffeinated water-solids mixture, so that they may absorb the lost solids.

How much goes back in? Not everything. That's why I've never much liked water-processed decaf, although the process has seen continual improvement. Once you remove everything that gives beans their flavor, they never taste the same. Nor is the water process always chemical-free, as advertised. The "Swiss Water Process," in which the caffeine is extracted by passing the water-solids solution through carbon filters, really is devoid of chemicals. Sometimes, though, in non-Swiss water processes, the caffeine is extracted from the water-solids solution with chemicals rather than with charcoal fiters. Chemical residues, albeit small amounts, have been found in water-processed decaffeinated beans in which the caffeine was extracted this way.

Sparkling Flavor

The most efficient chemical solvent, methylene chloride, is what people think they should avoid. Methylene chloride has been banned for use in hair sprays, because, in animal studies, it was shown to be dangerous when inhaled. But you don't get anywhere near that much when you drink chemically decaffeinated beans. Mice fed methylene chloride in drinking water at the equivalent of the amount in 4.4 million cups of decaffeinated coffee a day experienced no toxicological or carcinogenic response, although they did exhibit such responses when they inhaled it in much smaller quantities.

In 1985, the FDA declared the risk of methylene chloride in decaffeination to be so low "as to be essentially nonexistent." Methylene chloride evaporates at 180 degrees F. Beans are roasted to at least 350 degrees, and coffee is brewed at between 190 and 212 degrees. The amount of methylene chloride left in brewed coffee, then, is in parts per billion—less than is in the air of many cities. Even Michael Jacobson, the crusading leader of the consumer-advocate group Center for Science in the Public Interest, considers methylene chloride decaffeination a dead issue, saying that the universal use of caffeine is a matter of far greater concern than any chemical residues in decaffeinated coffee. Certainly, coffee decaffeinated using methylene chloride tastes best.

With worldwide sentiment among careful consumers veering away from anything using chemicals, the coffee industry has recognized a need for an alternative that offers flavor and body superior to what the water process generally yields. A preliminary answer was ethyl acetate, a chemical that occurs in tiny quantities in fruits like apples and bananas, which led its promoters to call decaffeination using it "natural process." Like methylene chloride, ethyl acetate is applied directly to beans and then evaporated. It is not nearly as specific to caffeine as methylene chloride, though, meaning that more of the flavor of the bean is carried away with the solvent.

A better answer might well be a new process using supercritical carbon dioxide. Carbon dioxide is, of course, a common gas, which beans emit in quantity soon after they are roasted. Blowing carbon dioxide through beans won't remove caffeine. But if enormous pressure is put on the gas, it turns into a fluid between liquid and gas; this pressurized "supercritical" fluid can pass through steamed coffee beans and take out the caffeine without removing other solids.

Its proponents say that, as a solvent, supercritical carbon dioxide is nearly as specific to caffeine as is methylene chloride, so that it removes the caffeine and nothing else. Best of all, the supercritical fluid vaporizes when its work is done and the pressure is eased—it turns into gas and dissipates, leaving not a trace.

If this process is so miraculous, why don't you see more beans decaffeinated using it? You do, without knowing it. So far, General Foods is the only company widely using the process in the United States, and its production capacity allows it to decaffeinate only its Sanka brand. Other beans decaffeinated with supercritical carbon dioxide haven't turned up in specialty shops because the plants where the process can take place require large investments, and the companies that can afford to build them have been interested in the mass market, not the specialty trade.

In 1993, I visited one of the handful of plants in the world that uses the supercritical carbon dioxide process; several companies use "carbon dioxide" in their publicity for their decaffeinated beans but have not made the large investment necessary to put the gas under sufficient pressure to render it truly supercritical. Located in the south of Italy and owned by a German company, the plant decaffeinates coffee for the widely distributed Caffè Hag brand. More important for the future of specialty coffee, the plant also decaffeinates quality beans for a small number of roasters and is trying to build a business in expensive, rare beans decaffeinated using its method.

I was impressed by how relatively unscathed the beans seemed after their high-pressure decaffeination—plumper and closer to their original greenish straw color than other decaffeinated beans, which are usually shriveled and brown from their long soaking and drying. And the taste, while still not up to that of the nondecaffeinated beans, was certainly better than water-processed beans and nearly as good as those decaffeinated with methylene chloride—still the gold standard. At one time an entrepreneur named Marc Sims tried to build a plant in the United States, but he eventually abandoned his plans when it became clear, he says, that the big roasters intended to stick with methylene chloride.

How Much Is Too Much?

Along with taste, the big question about decaffeinated coffee is how thoroughly decaffeinated it really is. "Regular, decaf—it's all caf," a woman once said dismissively when I offered her a choice of coffees after dinner. She was not entirely wrong. Advertisements for coffee that is "97 percent caffeine-free" can describe any coffee, with caffeine or decaffeinated, since the natural caffeine content of coffee varies from 1.1 to 2.6 percent. The FDA requires that coffee labeled "decaffeinated" have no more than 0.3 percent caffeine in brewed coffee. Coffee decaffeinated by a careful firm— such as KVW, near Hamburg, which uses methylene chloride and sends beans to a number of U.S. importers—has ten times less than this, 0.03 percent caffeine.

Not all plants are so scrupulous, because the law does not require them to be. Decaffeinated coffee can have 1 to 5 milligrams of caffeine per 5-ounce cup, depending on the process. This may sound like nothing, but I find that decaf often keeps me awake. I have not seen studies comparing caffeine levels of coffee brewed from the decaffeinated beans of different processing plants, but by experience I have found that the more expensive the decaffeinated beans, the more residual caffeine there seems to be. Mass-market decaf, on the other hand, has been processed with little concern for quality and much concern for the highest possible yield of caffeine for resale, and so it seems to be more trustworthy for someone who is extremely sensitive to caffeine. Perhaps when beans decaffeinated with the supercritical carbon dioxide method become more common, it will be easier to drink coffee after dinner. But for the moment herbal tea is the safest bet. Save what you love for the morning.

COMPARATIVE CAFFEINE

All values in milligrams (mg)

SUBSTANCE	TYPICAL	RANGE
1 cup brewed coffee (6 ounces)	100	77–150
1 shot espresso (2 ounces)	80	60–100
1 cup instant coffee (6 ounces)	70	20–130
1 cup decaffeinated coffee (6 ounces)	4	2–9
1 cup tea (6 ounces)	40	30–90
1 can caffeinated soda (12 ounces)	40	22–71
1 cup cocoa beverage (6 ounces)	7	2–10
1 glass chocolate milk (6 ounces)	4	2–7
1 milk chocolate bar (1.5 ounces)	10	2–10
1 dark chocolate bar (1.5 ounces)	30	5–35
1 tablet caffeine-containing cold remedy	25 or 50	25–50
1 tablet caffeine-containing pain reliever	32 or 65	32–65
1 tablet stimulant	100 or 200	75–350

Adapted from "Caffeine Pharmacology and Clinical Effects," by Roland R. Griffiths, Ph.D., Laura M. Juliano, Ph.D., and Allison L. Chausmer, Ph.D., from Principles of Addiction Medicine, *Third Edition (Graham, Schultz, Mayo-Smith, Ries, eds.). Chevy Chase, Md.: American Society of Addiction, 2003.*

9 Recipes

I LOVE COOKIES AND CAKES, but I find that there's something missing if I don't have a cup of coffee alongside them. Much as I have a sweet tooth, I don't like things too sweet. The bitterness of coffee offsets the sugar in the baked goods I crave.

Bitterness is not a flavor to shun, even though Americans have usually been afraid of it and prefer coffee with cream and sugar. I like bitter things, in moderation; bitter is, after all, one of the four basic flavor sensations the palate recognizes, along with sweet, salty and sour.

Like many bitter ingredients used subtly, coffee deepens flavors. Chefs often use secret ingredients to add mysterious depth and nuance to a dish, and coffee is one of them. In the classic American repertory, the most famous example of a savory dish with this hidden asset is red-eye gravy—a "divine elixir," as John Egerton writes in *Southern Food*, made of coffee mixed with the pan juices of hickory-smoked Southern country ham, a breakfast sauce to be served over ham with eggs.

Otherwise, coffee isn't usually paired with meat, except as a novelty. I tried a number of savory dishes from 1950s and 1960s coffee cookbooks that paired coffee with pork, veal and chicken and decided it wasn't surprising that the books are now out of print. Pork, the sweetest of the commonly consumed meats, was the most comfortable fit with coffee, in a sauce that also had capers. But a sauce made with coffee overwhelmed the veal cutlets I tried, and another did not make a persuasive match with chicken.

Coffee's most congenial companions, to my mind, are sugar and chocolate. Ever since Europeans discovered coffee, people have often described its taste as being like chocolate, and "mocha" has come to mean the combination of chocolate and coffee. Some combinations are mysteriously great: they release more flavors than either component has on its own. This is one of them.

The purest way to savor the marriage of chocolate and coffee is to enjoy a piece of chocolate with a cup of black, unsweetened espresso. In many Swiss and French restaurants, an after-dinner espresso or dark-roasted brewed coffee always comes with a square of bittersweet chocolate. A lusher experience is a creamy truffle with very strong coffee. The velvet smoothness of the chocolate melts immediately in the mouth to body temperature and, with a small sip of coffee, is warmed to a fragrant liquid.

Although nothing is as lock-and-key perfect with coffee as chocolate, a number of other flavors in desserts suit it nicely. One is the spice cardamom, which for centuries has been used to flavor brewed coffee in Turkey, Greece and throughout the Middle and Near East. In the recipes that follow, it appears in Cardamom Sugar Cookies (page 200) and a delicate Indian Rice Pudding (page 236). Orange zest is another excellent flavor pairing with coffee; ginger goes with coffee as well, in Ginger Perfects (page 196).

Nuts offer a slightly sweet, unctuous flavor that coffee balances superbly. Coffee's natural bitterness plays against their sweetness, and its acidity cuts the fat, the way vinegar does in a salad dressing—that's why coffee is such a natural with rich desserts. Hazelnuts and chocolate make nearly as great a combination with coffee as does plain chocolate. In my house, a special-occasion treat was Gianduia Cookies (page 202), chewy chocolate-hazelnut meringues (my mother's recipe called them "chocolate kisses"), which were served with coffee. Hazelnuts with coffee, too, are superb, as in Toasted Hazelnut Ice Cream (page 239). Peanut butter is, of course, classic with chocolate, at least in the United States, with its seemingly inborn taste for peanut butter; with coffee, the combination gains depth and becomes less cloying. Walnuts and especially pecans, America's finest nut, are also excellent against coffee.

For all its congeniality with dessert ingredients, coffee as a flavoring in baked goods can pose problems. Few baking recipes can accommodate enough brewed coffee to make a big impact on flavor without adversely affecting texture, even if the coffee is very strong. Although instant coffee is far from the ideal way to drink coffee, it is often the best way to inject a strong coffee flavor into a candy, cake or cookie. A home cook can make the equivalent of the kind of coffee essence a professional baker uses by mixing a much higher ratio of instant coffee granules to water than anyone would ever drink.

Added directly to baked goods, finely ground coffee lends both undiluted flavor and a texture that enhances a rich sweet. The ground coffee cuts the richness of Espresso-Hazelnut Russian Wedding Cakes (page 182), and it adds a pleasing cornmeal-like crunch. In other recipes, like Cappuccino Sandwiches (page 188) and Black and White Coffee Chip Cookies (page 190), ground coffee mixed into brewed or instant coffee gives more power to the flavor. In Mocha Brownies (page 214), the coffee punch comes from instant coffee granules dissolved in normal brewed coffee.

In all recipes calling for coffee, you might seriously consider using decaf—especially if you'll be serving a coffee-flavored sweet after dinner. Many of these recipes pack a lot of coffee: sampling the results in the afternoon sometimes gave me a jolt that lasted into the night.

Textures help determine what kind of coffee to serve with desserts. Just as the syrupy texture of espresso stands up to the powerful, mouth-filling richness of a piece of chocolate, a light-roast filter-brewed coffee is better for plain cakes, which beg for liquid to wash them down. Indispensable Snack Cake (page 220), a simple, un-iced one-layer cake, is a classic accompaniment to a milky cup of coffee.

A few recipes in this chapter can stand alone, substituting for a cup of coffee: Toasted Hazelnut Ice Cream and Cappuccino Mousse (page 237), for example, and Granita di Caffè (page 238), the marvelous shaved-ice dessert flavored with coffee, which Italians eat with tiny flat plastic shovels on summer days, topped with a cloud of whipped cream.

Then, of course, there is the hallowed tradition of dunking. Biscotti have replaced high-fat crullers as America's favorite thing to dunk. This chapter begins with three of my favorite biscotti. Like most of the other sweets that follow, however good they are on their own, they are made immeasurably better with coffee by their side.

Cookies and Bars

Cakes and Quick Breads

Puddings, Mousses and Ice Cream

Candies

Note: In most of the recipes, unsalted butter will give the best results. When salted butter is intended, it is listed simply as "butter."

Corby Kummer's Unbeatable Biscotti

I spent about two months perfecting this recipe, going through eighteen full batches before hitting on the exact formula. After I published the recipe, it generated a steady series of requests that still hasn't stopped a decade later. Bakers often tell me that no matter how many biscotti recipes they try, this is the one they stick with. They're not something I let myself make very often, though. I have absolutely no control over how many I eat.

These are the incredibly crisp kind that break in your mouth like glass and pack a roasted-almond punch, with no butter or other fat to distract you—just good, hard cookies and toasted nuts.

◆————————————————————————◆

1¼	cups whole almonds, blanched or unblanched
2	cups all-purpose flour
1	cup sugar
1	teaspoon baking soda
	Pinch of salt
3	large eggs
½	teaspoon pure vanilla extract

◆————————————————————————◆

1. Preheat the oven to 350 degrees F. Spread the almonds on a baking sheet and toast for 8 to 10 minutes, or until the smell permeates the air. Let cool. Reduce the oven temperature to 300 degrees. Line 2 baking sheets with parchment paper or foil, shiny side up. Arrange the oven racks to divide the oven into thirds.

2. **If using a mixer with a paddle attachment** (the dough is too stiff for a hand-held mixer): Stir together the dry ingredients in the mixer bowl. In a separate small bowl, lightly beat the eggs and vanilla. Blend the liquid ingredients into the dry ingredients at the lowest speed. The dough should cohere after a messy minute. It will be heavy and sticky. Pour in the nuts in 2 additions, beating just until the nuts begin to break. Turn out the dough onto a floured surface and fold it over itself 3 or 4 times to distribute the nuts. Let the dough rest for a minute or two.

If using a food processor: Whirl the eggs and vanilla for 5 seconds. Stir together the dry ingredients in a separate bowl and add them to the food processor, ½ cup at a time, pulsing about 5 times after each addition, until the dough almost incorporates the flour. After all the dry ingredients have been added, the dough will not quite form a ball. Add the nuts in 2 additions, pulsing 5 times after each one. The dough will still not cohere, and the nuts will not be well distributed. Turn out the pieces of dough onto a floured board, and with well-floured hands, fold the pieces over a dozen or so times in a rough kneading motion, or until the nuts are better distributed and the dough coheres. Let the dough rest for 5 minutes.

3. Divide the dough into 3 equal pieces. Working with lightly floured hands on a lightly floured surface, roll each piece into a rope about 1 inch wide and between 12 and 14 inches long. For dramatically larger biscotti, divide the dough in half and make 2 wider logs. Place the logs on the baking sheets, leaving at least 4 inches between the logs.

4. Bake for 40 minutes, reversing the sheets top to bottom halfway through the baking. Remove from the oven and cool for 5 minutes. Leave the oven on. Gently peel off the parchment paper or foil and place the bars on a cutting board. Using a sharp knife, cut the bars every ½ inch on the diagonal. Place the cookies, cut sides up, on the 2 baking sheets and toast in the oven for between 35 and 50 minutes, depending on how dark you like the cookies. Cool on a rack. Store the cookies in a container that admits air, which will keep them from softening.

YIELD: 4 DOZEN 3-INCH COOKIES
OR 2 DOZEN 6-INCH COOKIES

Unbeatable Chocolate Biscotti

This recipe strikes an ideal balance between the dry crunchiness of plain biscotti and a deep chocolate flavor that sets off the almonds beautifully without being cloying. It comes from Judith Barrett, a friend and writer on Italian food, who added to my original recipe and bakes these biscotti almost anytime she has guests. I can think of no finer accompaniment to a pot of coffee than a plate of plain and chocolate biscotti side by side. Be sure to have backup supplies.

1¼ cups unblanched whole almonds
1¾ cups all-purpose flour
⅓ cup unsweetened cocoa powder
2 tablespoons instant espresso or coffee powder
1 teaspoon baking soda
¼ teaspoon salt
4 ounces bittersweet or semisweet chocolate chips
3 large eggs
1 teaspoon pure vanilla extract
1 cup sugar

1. Preheat the oven to 350 degrees F. Spread the almonds on a baking sheet and toast for 10 minutes, or until the smell permeates the air. Transfer to a plate to cool.

2. Reduce the oven temperature to 300 degrees. Line 2 baking sheets with parchment paper or foil, shiny side up. Arrange the oven racks to divide the oven into thirds.

3. Sift together the flour, cocoa, espresso or coffee powder, baking soda and salt into a small bowl.

4. Place the chocolate chips in the bowl of a food processor fitted with a metal blade. Add ½ cup of the sifted dry ingredients and process for 20 to 30 seconds, or until the chocolate is very fine.

5. In a mixer bowl with a paddle attachment (the dough is too stiff for a hand-held mixer), beat the eggs and vanilla just to mix. On low speed, add the

processed-chocolate mixture, the remaining sifted dry ingredients and the sugar. Beat until the ingredients are combined, about a minute. The dough will be stiff. With the machine running on the lowest speed, add the almonds and mix well.

6. Turn out the dough onto a well-floured surface. Use a heavy spatula or pastry scraper to get all the dough out of the bowl. Flour your hands and form the dough into a brick shape. Divide the dough into 2 equal pieces and roll each piece into a log 12 inches long. Place each log diagonally on a baking sheet.

7. Bake for 50 minutes, reversing the sheets top to bottom halfway through the baking. Remove the baking sheets from the oven, but leave the oven on. Allow the baked dough to cool on the baking sheets for about 5 minutes; transfer to a cutting board. With a serrated knife, carefully cut the logs on an angle into cookies about ½ inch thick.

8. Transfer the cookies to the baking sheets, cut sides down, and bake again for 35 to 40 minutes, turning them over after 20 minutes, and again reversing the sheets top to bottom, until the cookies are completely dry and crisp.

9. Turn off the heat, open the oven door a crack and allow the cookies to come to room temperature. Store the cookies in a container that admits air, which will keep them from softening.

YIELD: 3 DOZEN COOKIES

Tozzetti da Compagnia
("Biscotti to Keep You Company")

In Italian these irresistible hazelnut biscotti are called *tozzetti*, literally "stubs," for their squat fingerlike shape. During the fall and winter, when hazelnuts from the orchards around Vetralla, near Rome, are fresh, Giulia Tondo, a local legend of a home baker who hones her skill on her grandchildren, keeps a constant supply of these tozzetti in the cookie jar. Giulia will tell you, correctly, that her tozzetti are better than everyone else's, and she'll even tell you her secrets. One is lard, which adds a barely identifiable and wonderful flavor; she uses it only if she knows who killed the pig and when, and she always combines it with butter. (If you can't find fresh lard or have no desire to look for it, butter will work fine.) Another is adding olive oil to soften the dough, which makes these cookies perfect for anyone who loves the toasted nuts and crunch of biscotti but doesn't want a strenuous jaw workout.

◆━━━━━━━━━━━━━━━━━━━━━━━━━━━━━━━━◆

1¼ cups whole hazelnuts (or whole almonds, if desired)
1¾ cups all-purpose flour
1 scant teaspoon baking powder
½ teaspoon salt
¼ cup (½ stick) butter, softened, or 2 tablespoons lard
    and 2 tablespoons butter
¾ cup sugar
3 large eggs, separated
1 tablespoon grated lemon zest
1 tablespoon olive oil or vegetable oil
2 teaspoons pure vanilla extract

◆━━━━━━━━━━━━━━━━━━━━━━━━━━━━━━━━◆

1. Preheat the oven to 350 degrees F. Set 2 racks in the oven to divide it into thirds. Roast the nuts on a baking sheet in the upper third of the oven for 10 to 15 minutes, or until the smell perfumes the air. To see if the nuts are toasted, cut one in half: it should be golden brown in the center. Leave the oven on and line 2 baking sheets with parchment paper or foil, shiny side up.

2. If using hazelnuts, place the nuts in a tea towel, cover with another towel and rub; the skins will slip off. Transfer the nuts to a plate or a bowl, shake out the towel and wrap the skinned nuts loosely in it. With the bottom of a heavy pot or a meat pounder, whack the nuts once or twice so they break into chunks—no smaller than half. Some nuts should remain whole. If using almonds, they need not be skinned and can remain whole.

3. Sift together the flour, baking powder and salt into a small bowl; set aside.

4. In the bowl of an electric mixer, cream the butter and lard, if using, for about a minute. Add the sugar and beat until well blended, about 2 minutes. With the mixer at medium speed, beat in the egg yolks, one at a time, waiting about 30 seconds until each is thoroughly incorporated. Beat for 3 to 5 minutes, or until pale. Beat in the lemon zest, oil and vanilla.

5. With the mixer running at its lowest speed, add the sifted dry ingredients in 3 or 4 additions; wait until they are incorporated before adding more. Beat in the nuts just until they are well distributed and begin to break up; the dough will be crumbly.

6. In a clean, dry medium bowl, beat 2 of the egg whites just until very soft peaks form and the whites still look wet. Fold the whites into the dough, mixing well. Don't worry about being delicate—you just need to make the dough come together. The dough will be slightly wet.

7. With floured hands on a floured surface, roll about a cup of dough at a time into logs ½ to ¾ inch in diameter. The length doesn't matter, and the logs do not have to be perfectly round. Slice into finger shapes, 2½ to 3 inches long. Place on the baking sheets 3 inches apart.

8. Bake for 15 minutes, or until set. Remove from the oven, brush with the remaining egg white, and return to the oven, reversing the baking sheets top to bottom. Bake for 10 minutes more, or until browned on both top and bottom. The undersides brown faster than the tops; watch carefully so they don't burn. Cool on a rack. Store at room temperature for a week or freeze for up to 4 months.

YIELD: 3 DOZEN COOKIES

Espresso-Hazelnut Russian Wedding Cakes

Usually called Russian tea cakes or Mexican wedding cakes, these crumbly spheres disappear in your mouth just as you're registering how incredibly good they are. Hazelnuts and espresso-grind coffee make them much more interesting than the plain walnut versions you've doubtless tried. The coffee amplifies the nuttiness and cuts the sweetness. These are by far the best version I've ever tasted of these dangerously good cookies.

◆———————————————————◆

Cookies
  1 cup whole hazelnuts
  2 tablespoons granulated sugar
  ½ cup (1 stick) butter, softened
  2 tablespoons confectioners' sugar
  1 teaspoon pure vanilla extract
  1 tablespoon finely ground coffee, preferably espresso
  1 cup all-purpose flour
Coating
  1 cup confectioners' sugar
  1 teaspoon finely ground coffee, preferably espresso

◆———————————————————◆

1. Preheat the oven to 350 degrees F, with a rack in the middle.

2. **Make the cookies:** Spread the hazelnuts on a baking sheet. Toast for 15 to 20 minutes, or until the smell permeates the air. To see if the nuts are toasted, cut one in half; it should be golden brown in the center. Remove from the oven; let cool slightly. To remove the skins, place the nuts in a tea towel, cover with another towel and rub; the skins will slip off.

3. Finely chop the hazelnuts in a food processor with a tablespoon of the granulated sugar. The sugar helps prevent the nuts from turning into paste. Set aside.

4. In a large bowl, with an electric mixer on medium speed, cream together the butter, the remaining tablespoon granulated sugar and the confectioners' sugar, about a minute. With the mixer running, add the vanilla and ground coffee and blend for about a minute more.

5. Add the flour and hazelnuts and mix well on medium speed. The dough should be firm and not sticky, and should form a ball around the mixing paddle or beaters.

6. Form the dough into two 12-inch-long logs. Cut each log into 24 even pieces. Roll each piece into a ball and place on an ungreased baking sheet (or a baking sheet lined with foil or parchment paper) about ½ inch apart.

7. Bake for 15 to 20 minutes, or until firm and lightly golden.

8. **Meanwhile, make the coating:** Combine the confectioners' sugar with the coffee in a small paper or plastic bag.

9. When the cookies are done, immediately place 3 or 4 cookies at a time in the bag and shake to coat. Cool on a rack. After the cookies are cool, repeat the coating procedure. Store in an airtight container for up to a week or freeze for up to 4 months.

YIELD: 4 DOZEN COOKIES

Praline Crisps

Browned butter is the secret of these lacy butterscotch toffee crisps, which shatter into crackling layers in the mouth, leaving a lovely caramel aftertaste.

◆━━━━━━━━━━━━━━━━━━━━━◆

- 1 cup (2 sticks) unsalted butter
- 1 cup all-purpose flour
- ½ teaspoon baking soda
- ¼ teaspoon salt
- 1½ cups firmly packed light brown sugar
- 1 large egg
- 2 teaspoons pure vanilla extract
- 2 cups chopped pecans

◆━━━━━━━━━━━━━━━━━━━━━◆

1. Melt the butter in a small saucepan over medium heat. Heat until it begins to brown and turns a deep golden color, about 5 minutes, stirring occasionally. Watch carefully to make sure it doesn't burn. Pour into a heatproof container to cool. Scrape out and discard the little dark brown flakes, but don't scrape out the darker film on the bottom. Refrigerate until solid, about 2 hours or overnight, or for an hour in the freezer.

2. Preheat the oven to 350 degrees F, with a rack in the middle. Lightly grease 2 baking sheets or line them with parchment paper.

3. Sift together the flour, baking soda and salt into a small bowl; set aside.

4. In a large bowl, with an electric mixer on medium speed, cream the browned butter for a minute. Add the brown sugar and cream until light and fluffy, about 2 minutes. With the mixer on low speed, blend in the egg and vanilla.

5. Gradually add the sifted dry ingredients and blend on low speed until smooth, about a minute.

6. Stir in the chopped pecans with a wooden spoon.

7. Drop the batter by rounded teaspoonfuls onto the baking sheet, about 2 inches apart; these cookies spread. Bake one sheet at a time for 10 to 12 minutes, or until firm and dark gold. Let the cookies cool on the baking sheet for a minute; remove and cool on wire racks. Store in an airtight container in layers, with wax paper between, for up to a week, or freeze for up to 4 months.

YIELD: 8 DOZEN 2-INCH COOKIES

Raya's Chocolate Wafers

These crunchy cookies, named for Lisë Stern's Aunt Raya, have a strong, not-sweet chocolate flavor. With raspberry jam sandwiched between them, they become elegant tea-party cookies.

◆————————————————————————————————◆

2½ cups all-purpose flour
2 teaspoons baking powder
½ cup (1 stick) unsalted butter, softened
1½ cups sugar
1 large egg, beaten
2 ounces unsweetened chocolate, melted and cooled
¼ teaspoon salt
¼ cup milk
½ cup raspberry jam (optional)

◆————————————————————————————————◆

1. Sift together the flour and baking powder into a small bowl; set aside.

2. In a large bowl, with an electric mixer on medium speed, cream together the butter and sugar for about 2 minutes. Add the egg, melted chocolate and salt. Blend thoroughly on medium speed, about a minute.

3. Add half of the flour mixture and mix well on medium speed. Add the milk and mix, then add the remaining flour and mix for about a minute.

4. Form the dough into 2 logs about 2 inches thick and 8 inches long. Wrap in plastic and refrigerate for several hours or overnight. (*The dough may be frozen for up to 3 months.*)

5. Preheat the oven to 350 degrees F, with a rack in the middle. Lightly grease 2 baking sheets or line them with parchment paper.

6. Remove the logs from the refrigerator, one at a time. Slice as thin as possible and place the rounds on the baking sheet, about ½ inch apart.

7. Bake one sheet at a time for 9 to 11 minutes, or until the cookies are firm. Remove from the baking sheet immediately and cool on wire racks.

8. When cool, you can eat the cookies plain or make sandwiches: Place ½ teaspoon raspberry jam on the underside of half the cookies and top with the remaining cookies. Store in an airtight container for up to a week or freeze, without the jam, for up to 9 months: they're good to have on hand for unexpected guests.

YIELD: 8 DOZEN COOKIES

Sesame Wafers

These are among my favorite wafer cookies, elegant semi-confections that get their deep flavor from browned sesame seeds.

⅔ cup sesame seeds
1 cup all-purpose flour
¼ teaspoon baking powder
¼ teaspoon salt
½ cup (1 stick) unsalted butter, softened
1¼ cups firmly packed light brown sugar
1 large egg
1 teaspoon pure vanilla extract

1. In a large skillet over medium heat, toast the sesame seeds, stirring occasionally, until they are golden brown. This can take about 15 to 20 minutes; turn the heat higher if it seems to be taking a while, but watch carefully—the seeds can suddenly burn. Set aside.

2. Preheat the oven to 325 degrees F, with a rack in the middle. Lightly grease 2 baking sheets or line them with parchment paper.

3. Sift together the flour, baking powder and salt into a small bowl; set aside.

4. In a large bowl, with an electric mixer on medium speed, cream together the butter and brown sugar until well blended, about 2 minutes.

5. Add the egg and vanilla and blend on medium speed, about a minute.

6. Add the flour mixture and mix well on medium speed, about a minute. Stir in the sesame seeds.

7. Drop the batter by scant teaspoonfuls onto the baking sheets, about 2 inches apart—the cookies will spread. Bake one sheet at a time for 15 to 20 minutes, or until firm. Let the cookies cool on the baking sheet for a minute, then remove and cool on wire racks. Store in an airtight container for up to a week or freeze for up to 6 months.

YIELD: 6 DOZEN COOKIES

Java Sticks

A simple butter cookie, subtly flavored with coffee and cocoa, from Flo Braker, which she kindly adapted from her book *Sweet Miniatures*. These are the shortbread sticks made with butter, festooned with chocolate and ground nuts at either end like a baton, that every bakery used to sell.

◆————————————————————————◆

1	cup (2 sticks) unsalted butter, softened
½	cup sugar
¼	cup unsweetened cocoa powder
2	teaspoons instant coffee powder, dissolved in 1 teaspoon pure vanilla extract
1¼	cups all-purpose flour
¼	cup walnuts, finely ground in a nut grinder
3	ounces semisweet chocolate, melted
	About 1½ cups chocolate sprinkles or ground walnuts

◆————————————————————————◆

1. Preheat the oven to 350 degrees F, with a rack in the lower third. Line a baking sheet with parchment paper.

2. In a large bowl, with an electric mixer on medium speed, cream the butter with the sugar. Beat in the cocoa powder and dissolved coffee. Add the flour and ground walnuts, blending well.

3. Place the dough in a pastry bag fitted with a ½-inch tip and pipe into 2-inch lengths onto the baking sheet. The dough will be stiff.

4. Bake for 10 to 15 minutes, or until the cookies are no longer shiny on the tops and the bottoms are just starting to brown. Cool on a rack.

5. Dip each end of the cookies into the melted chocolate and then into the sprinkles or nuts. Store in an airtight container.

YIELD: 6 DOZEN COOKIES

Cappuccino Sandwiches

The creamy coffee filling is so good that you should try these first as sandwiches. But the coffee-flavored wafers are wonderfully brittle and you'll also want to keep eating them alone.

After a day or two, the cinnamon becomes richer and more pronounced, so make these cookies ahead. If you intend to eat the wafers unfilled, cut them a bit thicker, as directed.

◆━━━━━━━━━━━━━━━━━━━━━━━━━━━━◆

Cookies
1½   cups all-purpose flour
½   teaspoon baking powder
¼   teaspoon baking soda
¼   teaspoon salt
¼–½ teaspoon ground cinnamon
½   cup (1 stick) unsalted butter, softened
½   cup firmly packed light brown sugar
½   cup sugar
2   tablespoons light corn syrup
1   large egg
2   teaspoons instant coffee powder, dissolved in
      1 tablespoon hot water
1½   teaspoons pure vanilla extract
1   teaspoon ground coffee (regular grind)
Creamy Coffee Filling
2   tablespoons (¼ stick) butter, softened
1   cup confectioners' sugar, sifted, or more as needed
1   teaspoon instant coffee powder, dissolved in
      4 teaspoons hot water

◆━━━━━━━━━━━━━━━━━━━━━━━━━━━━◆

1. **Make the cookies:** Sift together the flour, baking powder, baking soda, salt and desired amount of cinnamon into a small bowl; set aside.

2. In a large bowl, with an electric mixer on medium speed, cream together the butter and sugars until well blended, about 2 minutes. Add the corn syrup and mix well.

3. Add the egg, dissolved coffee and vanilla and mix until smooth on medium speed, about a minute.

4. Sprinkle the ground coffee over the batter, then pour on the flour mixture. Mix thoroughly on low speed, about 30 seconds.

5. Divide the dough into 2 logs, 12 inches long and about 1½ inches thick. Wrap in plastic and refrigerate overnight. *(The dough may be frozen at this point for up to 3 months. When you are ready to use it, defrost the dough for several hours in the refrigerator.)*

6. Preheat the oven to 350 degrees F, with a rack in the middle. Lightly grease a baking sheet or line with parchment paper.

7. Remove a roll of dough from the refrigerator. If making sandwich cookies, cut into ⅛-inch-thick slices. Place the slices on the baking sheet about ½ inch apart. If you are planning to serve the cookies plain, cut the dough into ¼-inch-thick slices and place about an inch apart on the baking sheet.

8. Bake for 10 to 12 minutes, or until firm and golden. Remove the cookies from the baking sheet immediately and cool on a wire rack.

9. **Meanwhile, make the filling:** Using an electric mixer or your fingers, blend together the butter and confectioners' sugar. With a fork, stir in the dissolved coffee. The filling should be of a spreadable consistency. If it is too thick, add a little water; if it is too thin, add more confectioners' sugar.

10. When the cookies are cool, turn them upside down. Using a knife, spread ¼ to ½ teaspoon of the filling on half the cookies. Press an unfrosted cookie on top. The filling will spread to the edge.

11. Place the cookies on a rack for a few hours to let the filling set. Store in an airtight container for up to a week or freeze, without the filling, for up to 3 months.

YIELD: 12 DOZEN UNFILLED COOKIES OR 6 DOZEN FILLED

Black and White Coffee Chip Cookies

These chocolate chip cookies have just the right crispness, with generous chunks of dark and white chocolate and flecks of ground coffee. The slightly higher than usual baking temperature deepens and unites the flavors, and ensures an uncompromisingly crisp texture.

1½ cups all-purpose flour
½ teaspoon baking soda
¼ teaspoon salt
⅔ cup unsalted butter, softened
½ cup firmly packed light brown sugar
½ cup sugar
1 large egg
1 teaspoon instant coffee powder, dissolved in
 1½ teaspoons pure vanilla extract
4 teaspoons ground coffee (regular grind)
½ cup semisweet chocolate chips
½ cup white chocolate chips

1. Preheat the oven to 375 degrees F, with a rack in the middle. Lightly grease 2 baking sheets or line them with parchment paper.

2. Sift together the flour, baking soda and salt into a small bowl; set aside.

3. In a large bowl, with an electric mixer on medium speed, cream together the butter and sugars until light and fluffy, scraping the bowl to make sure the batter is evenly blended.

4. Add the egg, instant coffee–vanilla mixture and ground coffee and blend on medium speed for about a minute.

5. Add the flour mixture and mix on medium speed until blended, about a minute.

6. Stir in both kinds of chocolate chips with a wooden spoon.

7. Drop the dough by scant tablespoonfuls onto the baking sheets, about 2 inches apart. Bake one sheet at a time for 12 to 14 minutes, or until the cookies are golden around the edges. Remove from the pan immediately and cool on wire racks. Store in an airtight container for up to a week or freeze for up to 4 months.

YIELD: ABOUT 40 COOKIES

Chock-Full-of-Nuts Chocolate Chip Cookies

This is Lisë Stern's favorite chocolate chip cookie recipe: nutty, crunchy and slightly chewy, based on variations of Neiman Marcus's or Mrs. Fields's chocolate chip cookies. "Though it may be blasphemy," says Lisë, who has been collecting chocolate chip recipes since she was twelve, "Toll House are not close to being the best recipe. They are too soft and cakey." The makers of M&M candies recently introduced a miniature, semisweet version of their traditional milk chocolate candies. These work much better in baking than the full-size milk chocolate ones and add another kind of crunch to the cookies. But regular chocolate chips work fine.

◆————————————————————————————◆

- 1 cup quick-cooking or old-fashioned rolled oats (not instant)
- ½ cup pecan halves, plus ½ cup coarsely chopped pecans
- 1 cup all-purpose flour
- ½ teaspoon baking soda
- ½ teaspoon baking powder
- ¼ teaspoon salt
- ½ cup (1 stick) unsalted butter, softened
- ½ cup firmly packed dark brown sugar
- ½ cup sugar
- 1 large egg
- 1½ teaspoons pure vanilla extract
- ¾ cup semisweet chocolate chips or M&Ms Semi-Sweet Chocolate Candies

◆————————————————————————————◆

1. Preheat the oven to 350 degrees F, with a rack in the middle. Lightly grease 2 baking sheets or line them with parchment paper.

2. Pulverize the oats and the ½ cup pecan halves in a blender or food processor.

3. Add the flour, baking soda, baking powder and salt and pulse to mix; set aside.

4. In a large bowl, with an electric mixer on medium speed, cream together the butter and sugars until light and fluffy, about a minute, scraping the bowl to make sure the batter is evenly blended.

5. Add the egg and vanilla and blend on medium speed.

6. Add the flour mixture and mix on medium speed until blended, about a minute.

7. Stir in the chocolate chips or candies and the ½ cup coarsely chopped pecans, using a wooden spoon.

8. Drop the batter by rounded tablespoonfuls onto the baking sheets, about 2 inches apart. Bake one sheet at a time for 10 to 12 minutes, or until the cookies are golden around the edges. Remove from the pan immediately and cool on a wire rack. Store in an airtight container for up to a week or freeze for up to 6 months.

YIELD: ABOUT 30 COOKIES

Mocha Chip Cookies

These darkly sophisticated cookies, neither too soft nor too crisp, are more potent than you might imagine. Of all the cookies offered here, they have the strongest mocha taste.

◆━━━━━━━━━━━━━━━━━━━━━━━━━━━━━━◆

1½ cups all-purpose flour
4   teaspoons unsweetened cocoa powder
½   teaspoon baking soda
¼   teaspoon salt
⅔   cup unsalted butter, softened
½   cup firmly packed light brown sugar
½   cup sugar
1   large egg
1½ teaspoons pure vanilla extract
¼   cup strong brewed coffee, mixed with 1 teaspoon
    instant coffee powder
2   teaspoons ground coffee (regular grind)
1   cup semisweet chocolate chips

◆━━━━━━━━━━━━━━━━━━━━━━━━━━━━━━◆

1. Preheat the oven to 350 degrees F, with a rack in the middle. Lightly grease 2 baking sheets or line them with parchment paper.

2. Sift together the flour, cocoa, baking soda and salt into a small bowl; set aside.

3. In a large bowl, with an electric mixer on medium speed, cream together the butter and sugars until light and fluffy, about 2 minutes. With the mixer running, add the egg and vanilla and mix thoroughly.

4. Add half the flour mixture and mix thoroughly on low speed. With the mixer running on low, add the brewed coffee and ground coffee.

5. Add the remaining flour mixture and mix thoroughly on low speed.

6. Stir in the chocolate chips with a wooden spoon.

7. Drop the dough by teaspoonfuls onto the baking sheet, about 2 inches apart. Bake one sheet at a time for 10 to 12 minutes, or until firm. Remove from the pan immediately and cool on a wire rack. Store in an airtight container for up to a week or freeze for up to 4 months.

Yield: 5 dozen 2-inch cookies

Orange-Ginger Chip Cookies

You'll swear that there's orange liqueur in these wide, crisp cookies, but the delightfully bittersweet orange flavor comes from zest and juice, with a welcome hint of ginger.

◆───────────────◆

1¼   cups all-purpose flour
¼   cup whole wheat flour
2½   teaspoons ground ginger
½   teaspoon baking soda
¼   teaspoon salt
⅔   cup unsalted butter, softened
½   cup firmly packed light brown sugar
½   cup sugar
1   large egg
1   teaspoon pure vanilla extract
1   tablespoon fresh orange juice
1   teaspoon orange zest
¾   cup semisweet chocolate chips

◆───────────────◆

1. Preheat the oven to 350 degrees F, with a rack in the middle. Lightly grease 2 baking sheets or line them with parchment paper.

2. Sift together the flours, ginger, baking soda and salt into a small bowl; set aside.

3. In a large bowl, with an electric mixer on medium speed, cream together the butter and sugars until light and fluffy, about 2 minutes.

4. Add the egg, vanilla, orange juice and orange zest and blend thoroughly on medium speed.

5. Add the flour mixture and mix on low speed until blended, about 30 seconds.

6. Stir in the chocolate chips with a wooden spoon.

7. Drop the dough by rounded teaspoonfuls onto the baking sheets, about 2 inches apart. Bake one sheet at a time for 12 to 15 minutes, or until the cookies are firm and golden around the edges. Remove from the pan immediately and cool on a wire rack. Store in an airtight container for up to a week or freeze for up to 4 months.

YIELD: ABOUT 4½ DOZEN COOKIES

Ginger Perfects

Lisë Stern, a champion cookie baker, calls these her all-time favorites, and I wouldn't dare argue. They're delicate, with a strong but not attacking taste of ginger, and a nice warm honey flavor behind them. The bit of allspice props up the ginger without dominating it. It took Lisë years to perfect the texture, which is thicker and less brittle than a wafer, somewhat chewy. No wonder she thinks they're perfect. The dough should be frozen overnight; plan accordingly.

2½ cups all-purpose flour
2 teaspoons baking soda
½ teaspoon ground allspice
¼ teaspoon salt
½ cup (1 stick) unsalted butter, softened
¼ cup (½ stick) margarine or vegetable shortening
½ cup firmly packed light brown sugar
½ cup sugar
¼ cup light, unsulfured molasses
¼ cup honey
1 large egg
1 teaspoon pure vanilla extract
1 tablespoon grated fresh ginger

1. Sift together the flour, baking soda, allspice and salt into a medium bowl; set aside.

2. In a large bowl, with an electric mixer on medium speed, cream together the butter, margarine or shortening and sugars until well blended, about 2 minutes.

3. With the mixer running, add, one at a time and blending well after each addition, the molasses, honey, egg, vanilla and grated ginger. Blend thoroughly, about a minute.

4. Add the flour mixture and mix well on medium speed, about a minute; the batter will be soft.

5. Chill the mixture in the refrigerator until firm, about an hour. Divide the dough into 4 portions and roll into logs about 1½ inches thick and 8 inches

long. Wrap in plastic and freeze overnight. *(The dough may be frozen, wrapped in foil, for up to 3 months.)*

6. Preheat the oven to 350 degrees F, with a rack in the middle. Lightly grease 2 baking sheets or line them with parchment paper.

7. Remove the logs from the freezer, one at a time. Slice into ¼-inch-thick rounds and place on the baking sheets, about an inch apart.

8. Bake one sheet at a time for 12 to 14 minutes, or until the cookies are firm and dark gold. Remove from the baking sheet immediately and cool on wire racks. Store in an airtight container for up to 2 weeks or freeze for up to 3 months.

YIELD: 10 DOZEN COOKIES

Toasted Almond–Lemon Slices

Coarsely chopped almonds stud these thin cookies, which combine many of the appealing qualities of biscotti—they're nutty and crunchy —with the richness of butter cookies. A tart lemon glaze sets them off perfectly and gives you a chance to show your decorative powers: the half-rounds can be iced to look like sliced lemons.

Cookies

1 cup whole almonds, blanched or unblanched

2 tablespoons plus 1 teaspoon granulated sugar

½ cup (1 stick) unsalted butter, softened

2 tablespoons confectioners' sugar

2 teaspoons lemon extract

Grated zest of 2 lemons

2 tablespoons fresh lemon juice

1 cup all-purpose flour

Coating

1 cup confectioners' sugar

Lemon Icing

½ cup confectioners' sugar, or more as needed

About 4 teaspoons fresh lemon juice

1. **Make the cookies:** Preheat the oven to 350 degrees F. Spread the almonds on a baking sheet and toast until the smell permeates the air, 10 to 15 minutes. Let cool completely. When cool, coarsely chop the almonds in a food processor with a teaspoon of the granulated sugar, using the pulse button.

2. In a large bowl, with an electric mixer on medium speed, cream together the butter, the remaining 2 tablespoons granulated sugar and the confectioners' sugar until well blended, about 2 minutes. Add the lemon extract and zest and blend on medium speed.

3. With the mixer running, gradually add the lemon juice and blend.

4. Add the flour and almonds and mix well on medium speed; the dough will be slightly soft but not sticky.

5. Form the dough into a 9-inch-long log, about 1¾ inches in diameter, and wrap in plastic. Chill the mixture in the refrigerator until firm, about an hour, or 20 minutes in the freezer.

6. Preheat the oven to 350 degrees F, with a rack in the middle.

7. Remove the log of dough from the refrigerator. Cut it into thirds, then cut each third in half horizontally. Slice each half-cylinder into ¼-inch-thick slices and place on an ungreased baking sheet about ½ inch apart.

8. Bake for 15 to 20 minutes, or until firm and lightly golden around the edges.

9. **Make the coating:** Have the 1 cup confectioners' sugar ready in a shallow bowl. As soon as you remove the cookies from the oven, gently roll them in the confectioners' sugar to coat, then cool on wire racks.

10. **While the cookies cool, make the icing:** Combine the confectioners' sugar with the lemon juice in a small bowl. Stir with a fork until smooth. The icing should drizzle from the fork. If it is too thick, add more lemon juice; if too thin, add more confectioners' sugar.

11. When the cookies are cool, drizzle them with the lemon icing. Or to decorate the cookies like sliced lemons, spoon the icing into a pastry bag fitted with a very narrow tip or into a small plastic bag and make a tiny snip at one corner. Outline a fan pattern on each cookie to resemble a lemon section. Let the icing set for at least an hour before storing. Store in an airtight container, with wax paper between the layers, for up to a week, or freeze, unfrosted, for up to 3 months.

YIELD: 6 DOZEN COOKIES

Cardamom Sugar Cookies

These thin cookies flavored with orange zest are wonderfully crisp.
Honey and brown sugar give them a nuanced, dark sweetness.

◆━━━━━━━━━━━━━━━━━━━━━━━━━━━━━━━━━━━━━◆

3¾ cups all-purpose flour
2 teaspoons baking soda
½ teaspoon ground cardamom
¼ teaspoon salt
1 cup (2 sticks) unsalted butter, softened
1 cup sugar
½ cup firmly packed light brown sugar
¼ cup honey
1 large egg
2 teaspoons pure vanilla extract
1 tablespoon grated orange zest (from 1 orange)

◆━━━━━━━━━━━━━━━━━━━━━━━━━━━━━━━━━━━━━◆

1. Sift together the flour, baking soda, cardamom and salt into a medium bowl; set aside.

2. In a large bowl, with an electric mixer on medium speed, cream to0gether the butter and sugars until well blended. Blend in the honey.

3. Add the egg, vanilla and orange zest, and blend on medium speed for about a minute.

4. Add the flour mixture and mix well on medium speed, about a minute.

5. Divide the dough into 3 portions and form into flat disks, about ¾ inch thick. Wrap in plastic and refrigerate at least 3 hours or overnight.

6. Preheat the oven to 350 degrees F, with a rack in the middle. Lightly grease 2 baking sheets or line with parchment paper.

7. Remove a disk from the refrigerator. Roll out the dough on a lightly floured surface until ⅛ inch thick. (The dough is easy to work with and flexible.) Cut into the desired shapes and place about an inch apart on the baking sheet.

8. Bake one sheet at a time for 10 to 12 minutes, until the cookies are firm and light gold around the edges. (You can roll out and cut the dough for the next sheet while the first batch bakes.) Remove the cookies from the pan immediately and cool on a wire rack. Store in an airtight container for up to 2 weeks or freeze for up to 9 months.

YIELD: ABOUT 9 DOZEN 2-INCH COOKIES

Coffee Clouds

Simple and fast, these meringues are just the thing when you don't think you're hungry but feel the need for something sweet to eat with coffee. They're especially appropriate after dessert, when they are elegant beside a cup of espresso. You might want to use decaf in them if you're serving these late at night; one cookie is never enough.

Make these cookies on a dry day.

---

2 large egg whites
⅛ teaspoon salt
⅛ teaspoon cream of tartar
½ cup sugar
2 teaspoons ground coffee (regular grind)
1 teaspoon instant coffee powder, dissolved in
   2 teaspoons Kahlúa or other coffee liqueur
½ teaspoon pure vanilla extract

---

1. Preheat the oven to 300 degrees F, with a rack in the middle. Lightly grease 2 baking sheets or line them with parchment paper.

2. With an electric mixer on medium speed (use the whisk attachment if using a standing mixer), whisk the egg whites with the salt and cream of tartar until soft peaks form.

3. With the mixer running, gradually add the sugar, about a tablespoon at a time.

4. Scrape the sides of the bowl. Add the ground coffee, instant coffee–liqueur mixture and vanilla. Whisk on medium speed a few seconds, just until incorporated.

5. Drop the batter onto the baking sheets by scant teaspoonfuls, about an inch apart.

6. Bake one sheet at a time for 40 minutes, until the cookies are firm. Let cool completely on the sheet before removing. Store in an airtight container for up to 2 weeks or freeze for up to 4 months.

YIELD: 4 DOZEN COOKIES

Gianduia Cookies

These chewy meringue cookies are based on my favorite flavor combination—hazelnuts and chocolate, called *gianduia* in northern Italy—and on my favorite childhood cookie, one my mother made for special occasions (her recipe called them "Chocolate Kisses"). Some people like them crisp, with an additional egg white, as in the variation at the end of the recipe. But I like them chewy in the middle and slightly crisp around the edges, with the surprise of toasted hazelnut chunks every other bite.

It's best to make these cookies on a dry day: humidity is not good for meringues.

◆————————————————————————————◆

1 cup whole hazelnuts
3 large egg whites
¾ cup sugar
1 teaspoon pure vanilla extract
3 ounces semisweet chocolate, melted and cooled
3 tablespoons unsweetened cocoa powder

◆————————————————————————————◆

1. Preheat the oven to 350 degrees F.

2. Spread the hazelnuts on a baking sheet. Toast for 15 to 20 minutes, or until the smell permeates the air. To see if the nuts are toasted, cut one in half; it should be golden brown in the center. Remove from the oven; let cool slightly. To remove the skins, place the nuts on a tea towel, cover with another towel and rub; the skins will slip off. Finely chop ⅓ cup of the nuts.

3. Reduce the oven heat to 325 degrees, with a rack in the middle. Lightly grease 2 baking sheets or line them with parchment paper.

4. In a large bowl, with an electric mixer on medium speed (use the whisk attachment on a standing mixer), beat the egg whites until soft peaks form.

5. With the mixer running, gradually add the sugar. Scrape the sides of the bowl, add the vanilla and whisk just until incorporated.

6. Add the melted chocolate and whisk until incorporated. Stir in the cocoa until mixed, then whisk for a few seconds on medium speed.

7. Using a rubber spatula, stir in the chopped and whole hazelnuts until incorporated.

8. Drop the batter onto the baking sheet by tablespoonfuls, about 2 inches apart.

9. Bake one sheet at a time for 15 to 20 minutes, or until the cookies are firm. Let cool completely on the baking sheet before removing. Store in an airtight container for up to a week or freeze for up to 4 months.

Variation: For a crisper, less chewy cookie, use 4 egg whites.

YIELD: 40 COOKIES

Mocha Marmalade Moons

You'll taste the lemon rind in the filling of these flaky, adult cookies and wonder what the alluring darker flavors are, but they remain mysterious. In fact, they're orange marmalade, unsweetened chocolate and coffee liqueur. The tender crust is inspired by both the original *Joy of Cooking* and Flo Braker's never-fail cream cheese dough from *The Simple Art of Perfect Baking,* with the addition of lemon rind and vanilla. The pastry must chill overnight, so plan ahead.

◆━━━━━━━━━━━━━━━━━━━━━━━━━━━━◆

Cream Cheese Pastry
½ cup (1 stick) unsalted butter, softened
4 ounces cream cheese, softened
¾ teaspoon grated lemon zest
½ teaspoon pure vanilla extract
1 cup all-purpose flour
¼ teaspoon salt

Filling
½ cup orange marmalade
1 ounce unsweetened chocolate, grated
1 tablespoon ground coffee (regular grind)
2 tablespoons Kahlúa or other coffee liqueur
¾ teaspoon grated lemon zest
1 tablespoon fresh lemon juice

◆━━━━━━━━━━━━━━━━━━━━━━━━━━━━◆

1. **Make the pastry:** In a large bowl, with an electric mixer on medium speed, blend the butter and cream cheese until smooth, about 2 minutes. Add the lemon zest and vanilla and blend until incorporated, about 30 seconds.

2. Add the flour and salt and blend just until the dough comes together, about 30 seconds.

3. Form the dough into 2 disks, wrap in plastic and chill overnight.

4. **Make the filling:** In a small bowl, combine all the ingredients and blend.

5. Preheat the oven to 400 degrees F, with a rack in the middle. Lightly grease a baking sheet or line it with parchment paper.

6. Remove the dough from the refrigerator and roll out each disk on a

lightly floured surface until about ⅛ inch thick. Cut the dough into 2½-inch circles.

7. Place a teaspoon of filling on one half of each circle. Moisten the edge and fold in half, forming a half-moon. Use a fork to crimp the edges firmly, or these cookies will spring open as they bake. Place the cookies on the baking sheet.

8. Bake for 20 to 25 minutes, or until the edges of the cookies are golden brown. Remove the cookies from the baking sheet immediately and cool on wire racks. These cookies are best eaten the day they are made.

YIELD: 2 DOZEN COOKIES

Apricot-Walnut Strudel Cookies

These strudel cookies are filled with a sweet mixture of apricot jam, walnuts and golden and dark raisins. Lisë Stern's grandmother-in-law Nancy Robbins made them for every family gathering.

◆━━━━━━━━━━━━━━━◆

Pastry
- ½ cup sour cream
- ¼ cup (½ stick) unsalted butter, softened
- 1 cup all-purpose flour
- ¼ teaspoon salt

Filling
- ⅔ cup apricot jam
- ⅔ cup chopped walnuts
- 2 tablespoons raisins
- 2 tablespoons golden raisins

◆━━━━━━━━━━━━━━━◆

1. **Make the pastry:** With an electric mixer on medium speed, blend the sour cream and butter until smooth, about 2 minutes. Add the flour and salt and blend until the dough comes together, about 30 seconds.

2. Form the dough into 2 disks, wrap in plastic and chill overnight.

3. Remove the dough from the refrigerator and let soften slightly, about 10 minutes. Preheat the oven to 350 degrees F, with a rack in the middle. Lightly grease a baking sheet.

4. On a lightly floured surface, roll out each disk to a circle about 9 to 10 inches in diameter and less than ⅛ inch thick.

5. **Make the filling:** Spread ⅓ cup apricot jam over the surface of a disk, leaving a ¼-inch border around the edges. Sprinkle ⅓ cup of the walnuts, a tablespoon of the raisins and a tablespoon of the golden raisins over the jam.

6. Roll up the dough jelly-roll fashion, pinching the ends together. Carefully lift the roll with your hands and transfer to the baking sheet. With a sharp knife, slice the roll halfway through into about 12 sections.

7. Repeat the procedure with the remaining dough and filling.

8. Bake for 40 to 45 minutes, or until golden brown. Cool on the baking sheet for 5 minutes. Cut the slices through; cool completely on the sheet. Store in an airtight container for up to a week or freeze for several months.

YIELD: 2 DOZEN COOKIES

Coffee Amaretti

I love amaretti—Italian macaroons, chewy with almond paste—but I usually have a limited capacity for them because they're so sweet. In these, however, the ground coffee and coffee liqueur cut the sweetness. Note that they require a cookie press or a pastry tube, which makes it easy to produce dozens at a time. To make them kosher for Passover, eliminate the flour and add 2 more tablespoons of almonds.

◆————————————————————————◆

7	ounces almond paste
½	cup sugar
¼	cup almonds, blanched or unblanched
2	large egg whites
1	teaspoon pure vanilla extract
1	teaspoon Kahlúa or other coffee liqueur
1	tablespoon all-purpose flour
2	teaspoons ground coffee (regular grind)
	Chocolate-covered coffee beans, for decoration (optional)

◆————————————————————————◆

1. Preheat the oven to 300 degrees F, with a rack in the middle. Lightly grease 2 baking sheets or line them with parchment paper.

2. In a food processor, combine the almond paste, sugar and almonds. Pulse until blended.

3. Add the egg whites and process until blended. With the machine running, add the vanilla and coffee liqueur.

4. Add the flour and ground coffee and pulse until blended; the batter will be sticky.

5. Place the batter in a cookie press or a pastry bag fitted with a ¼-inch star tip. Form the cookies into 1-inch stars on the baking sheets, about an inch apart. Alternatively, use a spoon to drop the batter by scant ½ teaspoonfuls onto the baking sheet. If desired, top with a chocolate-covered coffee bean, pressing down slightly.

6. Bake one sheet at a time for 25 to 30 minutes, or until firm. Let cool completely on the baking sheet before removing. Store in an airtight container for up to 2 weeks or freeze for up to 6 months.

YIELD: 7 DOZEN COOKIES

Rosemary Zaletti

Nothing pleases me more than the nutty crunch of cornmeal in baked goods. Italians regularly eat butter-cornmeal cookies like these; the rosemary is a Tuscan touch that makes the cookies both refined and rustic. These are great, unusual cookies that have proved to be enduringly popular.

◆————————————————————◆

1⅓ cups all-purpose flour
1 cup yellow cornmeal
¾ teaspoon dried rosemary
¼ teaspoon baking powder
¼ teaspoon salt
¾ cup (1½ sticks) unsalted butter, softened
¾ cup sugar
1 large egg
1½ teaspoons pure vanilla extract

◆————————————————————◆

1. Preheat the oven to 375 degrees F, with a rack in the middle. Lightly grease 2 baking sheets or line them with parchment paper.

2. In a small bowl, stir together the flour, cornmeal, rosemary, baking powder and salt; set aside.

3. In a large bowl, with an electric mixer on medium speed, cream together the butter and sugar until well blended, about 2 minutes.

4. With the mixer running, add the egg and vanilla. Blend thoroughly, about a minute.

5. Add the flour mixture and mix well on medium speed, about a minute; the batter will be firm but pliable.

6. You can shape the dough in two ways. Pinch off about a teaspoon of dough for each cookie. Either roll into a snake and make into an S shape, or roll into a ball and flatten with the bottom of a glass. For a sweeter cookie, dip the glass in sugar before flattening the dough, or dip the glass in cornmeal. The cookies should be very thin, about ⅛ inch thick. Place the cookies about an inch apart on the baking sheets.

7. Bake one sheet at a time for 10 to 15 minutes, or until firm and light gold around the edges. Remove the cookies from the baking sheet immediately and cool on wire racks. Store in an airtight container for up to a month or freeze for up to 6 months.

YIELD: 9 DOZEN COOKIES

Chocolate Peanut Butter Cups

Even if these look and sound like something for children, everyone loves the combination of peanut butter, chocolate and graham crackers. Sweetened condensed milk lends sugar and caramel flavors and also ensures that these will keep at room temperature for many days.

◆————————————————————◆

Chocolate Layer

1⅓ cups graham cracker crumbs

4 ounces semisweet chocolate, melted

¾ cup sweetened condensed milk

1 teaspoon pure vanilla extract

Peanut Butter Layer

⅔ cup graham cracker crumbs

½ teaspoon pure vanilla extract

½ cup sweetened condensed milk

⅓ cup smooth peanut butter

◆————————————————————◆

1. Preheat the oven to 350 degrees F, with a rack in the middle. Lightly grease two 12-cup (or one 24-cup) mini-muffin tins or lightly grease a baking sheet or line it with parchment paper.

2. **Make the chocolate layer:** In a medium bowl, with an electric mixer on medium speed, mix all the ingredients until well blended; set aside.

3. **Make the peanut butter layer:** In a small bowl, with an electric mixer on medium speed, mix all the ingredients until well blended; set aside.

4. Divide the chocolate mixture among the muffin cups. Press an indentation in the center of each, pushing the chocolate dough slightly up the sides of the cups. Alternatively, if using a baking sheet, divide the chocolate mixture into 24 pieces. Roll each piece into a ball and place them on the baking sheet about an inch apart. Press an indentation into the center of each ball.

5. Form the peanut butter mixture into 24 balls and drop into the chocolate indentations. Flatten slightly.

6. Bake for 25 to 30 minutes, or until the peanut butter cups are firm. Cool in the pan on a wire rack, then remove from the pan. Store in an airtight container for up to a week or freeze for up to 3 months.

YIELD: 2 DOZEN COOKIES

Congo Bars

These are similar to blondies—sweet, dense bar cookies with chocolate chips and walnuts. The recipe is from Flo Braker, author of *The Simple Art of Perfect Baking,* who developed it to meet the requests of friends. It's simple and pleasing.

⅔ cup unsalted butter, melted and cooled

2⅓ cups firmly packed light brown sugar (1 pound)

3 large eggs

2¾ cups all-purpose flour

2½ teaspoons baking powder

½ teaspoon salt

1 cup semisweet chocolate chips

1 cup chopped walnuts

1. Preheat the oven to 325 degrees F, with a rack in the lower third. Generously grease a 10-by-15-inch pan.

2. In a large bowl, using a mixer at low speed, blend the melted butter, brown sugar and eggs just until combined.

3. Sift the flour, baking powder and salt into another bowl and add to the egg mixture. Using a wooden spoon, stir in the chocolate chips and walnuts.

4. Spread the dough in the pan, patting it out with wet fingertips to prevent sticking. Bake for 30 to 35 minutes; it will still look soft. Cool in the pan on a wire rack. Cut while still warm into 25 bars. Store in an airtight container for up to 3 days or freeze for up to 2 weeks.

YIELD: 25 BARS

Marbled Brownie Wedges

Brownies that put on the dog, these are as elegant as a cake and as rich as brownies. The crust, a confection in itself, is given punch by ground coffee, and the marbled brownies subtly echo the coffee flavor while delivering the traditional chocolate and walnuts.

◆————————————————————————————◆

Walnut Crust
⅔ cup all-purpose flour
⅓ cup firmly packed light brown sugar
⅔ cup walnuts
1 teaspoon ground coffee (regular grind)
⅛ teaspoon salt
⅓ cup (5⅓ tablespoons) unsalted butter, chilled and cut into pieces

Brownie Filling
6 tablespoons (¾ stick) unsalted butter, softened
½ cup sugar
⅓ cup firmly packed light brown sugar
2 large eggs
1 tablespoon instant coffee powder, dissolved in 2 teaspoons pure vanilla extract
½ teaspoon baking powder
¼ teaspoon salt
1 cup all-purpose flour
½ cup coarsely chopped walnuts
1 ounce unsweetened chocolate, melted and cooled

◆————————————————————————————◆

1. Preheat the oven to 350 degrees F, with a rack in the middle. Lightly grease a 10-inch springform pan.

2. **Make the crust:** In the bowl of a food processor, combine the flour, brown sugar, walnuts, ground coffee and salt. Pulse until the nuts are finely chopped.

3. Add the butter and pulse until it is incorporated; the mixture should be crumbly, but it will hold together when pressed.

4. Place the crust crumbs in the pan and press down to form a uniform crust; set aside.

5. **Make the filling:** In a large bowl, with an electric mixer on medium speed, beat the butter with the sugars until light and fluffy, about 2 minutes.

6. Add the eggs, one at a time, beating until smooth on medium speed, about 30 seconds. Add the instant coffee–vanilla mixture and blend on medium speed for about a minute.

7. Sprinkle the baking powder and salt over the batter, then sprinkle the flour over. On low speed, mix until just combined. Using a wooden spoon, stir in the walnuts.

8. Pour two-thirds of the batter onto the crust and spread it in a thin layer to the edges.

9. Add the melted chocolate to the remaining third of the batter and mix thoroughly. Drop spoonfuls of the chocolate batter on top of the coffee batter. Use a knife to swirl the batter around and smooth the surface.

10. Bake for 30 to 35 minutes, or until set. Cool in the pan on a wire rack, remove the sides of the pan and cut into wedges. Refrigerate in an airtight container for up to a week or freeze, wrapped in plastic, then in foil, for up to 6 months.

YIELD: 16 WEDGES

Mocha Brownies

Brownies are by definition sweet, but the sweetness of these is moderated by the strong dose of coffee flavor. Because of the strength of the coffee and the relatively small amount of sugar, these are my favorite brownies.

◆——◆

3 tablespoons unsalted butter

2 ounces milk chocolate

2 large eggs

½ cup plus 2 tablespoons firmly packed light brown sugar

1 teaspoon instant coffee powder, dissolved in 1 teaspoon pure vanilla extract

¼ cup brewed coffee

1 tablespoon ground coffee (regular grind)

½ cup all-purpose flour

¼ teaspoon salt

◆——◆

1. Preheat the oven to 350 degrees F, with a rack in the middle. Lightly grease an 8-inch square pan.

2. In the top of a double boiler over simmering water, or in a glass bowl in a microwave oven, melt the butter and chocolate together. Stir until smooth; set aside to cool.

3. In a large bowl, with an electric mixer on medium speed, beat the eggs for a minute, then add the brown sugar and instant coffee–vanilla mixture and beat for 2 minutes. Stir in the brewed coffee and ground coffee.

4. Add the chocolate mixture and mix thoroughly on medium speed.

5. Blend in the flour and salt just until incorporated, about 30 seconds on low speed. Pour into the pan.

6. Bake for 20 to 25 minutes, or until firm. Cool in the pan on a wire rack for 15 minutes, then cut into 16 squares. Refrigerate in an airtight container for up to a week or freeze, wrapped in plastic wrap, then in foil, for up to 6 months.

YIELD: 16 BROWNIES

Pecan Vanilla Diamonds

Amazingly fast to throw together and always popular, these bar cookies are similar to shortbread, but their higher sugar content gives them a crisper texture after they cool. These go perfectly with fruit or ice cream.

1   cup (2 sticks) butter, softened
¾   cup sugar
¼   cup firmly packed light brown sugar
1   tablespoon pure vanilla extract
2   cups all-purpose flour
1   cup chopped pecans
    About 1½ cups pecan halves, for decoration

1. Preheat the oven to 375 degrees F, with a rack in the middle.

2. In a large bowl, with an electric mixer on medium speed, cream the butter with the sugars just until blended, about a minute. Blend in the vanilla.

3. Add the flour and blend on medium speed, about a minute. Stir in the chopped pecans.

4. Press the dough into an ungreased 11-by-17-inch pan; do not line the pan with foil or parchment paper; these cookies must be cut in the pan.

5. Score the dough into diamonds, without cutting all the way through: Cut diagonally from the lower left corner to the upper right corner. Cut 5 parallel lines on either side of this line for a total of 11 lines. Then cut diagonally from the upper left to the lower right and cut 5 parallel lines on either side again. Press a pecan half into each full diamond. You can use broken pecan pieces to decorate the triangles that are left along the edges of the pan.

6. Bake for 20 to 25 minutes, or until golden; the edges will be puffy and higher than the centers.

7. Let cool for 2 minutes, then cut along the scored lines while the cookies are still warm and soft. As they cool, the cookies become crisp and brittle. After slicing, let cool in the pan for another 5 minutes, then remove to wire racks to finish cooling. Store in an airtight container for up to a week or freeze for up to 6 months.

YIELD: ABOUT 44 DIAMONDS,
PLUS ADDITIONAL TRIANGULAR COOKIE PIECES

Coffee Pecan-Pie Squares

These squares are much easier to eat than pie. The filling won't run, and the ratio of toasted pecans on top to the filling is generous enough that you won't be tempted to pick off the nuts first. Flecks of ground coffee in the filling cut the sweetness and, to my mind, greatly improve a traditional favorite.

◆──◆

Pastry Crust
- 1 cup all-purpose flour
- ¼ cup firmly packed light brown sugar
- ¼ teaspoon salt
- ⅓ cup (5⅓ tablespoons) unsalted butter, chilled and cut into pieces
- 2 tablespoons plain yogurt

Pecan Filling
- 3 tablespoons unsalted butter, softened
- ⅓ cup firmly packed light brown sugar
- ⅓ cup sugar
- ⅓ cup light corn syrup
- 2 large eggs
- 1 tablespoon Kahlúa or other coffee liqueur
- 2½ teaspoons ground coffee (regular grind)
- 2 cups pecan halves
- ½ cup chopped pecans

◆──◆

1. Preheat the oven to 350 degrees F, with a rack in the middle. Lightly grease a 9-by-13-inch pan.

2. **Make the crust:** In a food processor, combine the flour, brown sugar and salt. Pulse to blend.

3. Add the butter pieces and pulse until the mixture is the consistency of cornmeal. With the machine running, add the yogurt and pulse just until incorporated, about 10 seconds. The mixture will be crumbly, but will hold together when pressed.

4. Press the crust into the pan. Pierce the surface evenly with a fork.

5. Bake for 15 to 20 minutes, or until the edges of the crust turn light brown; leave the oven on.

6. **Make the filling:** In a large bowl, with an electric mixer on medium speed, cream the butter with the sugars until well blended, about 2 minutes. Blend in the corn syrup.

7. Add the eggs, one at a time, blending well after each one. Add the coffee liqueur and ground coffee and beat on medium speed for a minute. With a wooden spoon, stir in the pecan halves and chopped pecans.

8. Pour the filling over the prebaked crust. Use a rubber spatula to spread the filling to the edges.

9. Bake for 25 minutes, or until the filling is browned and somewhat firm. Cool on a wire rack before cutting into 32 squares. Larger squares are easier to cut, but these cookies are rich, so smaller squares are better. Refrigerate in an airtight container for up to a week.

YIELD: 32 SMALL SQUARES

Raspberry Strata Bars

These rich and delicious squares, a combination of coffee cake, granola and jam tart, from the dessert authority Flo Braker can be made with almost any kind of jam you like, or even with chopped chocolate.

Streusel

1¼ cups old-fashioned or quick-cooking rolled oats (not instant)

1 cup all-purpose flour

1 cup firmly packed brown sugar

1 cup chopped walnuts

1¼ teaspoons baking powder

¾ teaspoon ground cinnamon

⅛ teaspoon salt

½ cup plus 2 tablespoons (1¼ sticks) unsalted butter, chilled and cut into ¼-inch-thick slices

Bar Dough

1½ cups chopped walnuts

1 cup all-purpose flour

⅔ cup sugar

½ teaspoon ground cinnamon

¼ teaspoon salt

⅛ teaspoon baking powder

½ cup plus 2 tablespoons (1¼ sticks) unsalted butter, chilled and cut into ¼-inch-thick slices

1 large egg

Filling and Topping

1 cup seedless raspberry jam, plus additional, if desired Confectioners' sugar (optional)

1. **Make the streusel:** In a large bowl with an electric mixer on low speed, preferably with the paddle attachment, combine the oats, flour, brown sugar, walnuts, baking powder, cinnamon and salt. Add the butter and mix until the topping has a crumbly granola-like consistency.

2. Preheat the oven to 350 degrees F, with a rack in the lower third.

3. **Make the dough:** In a food processor, process the nuts, flour, sugar, cinnamon, salt and baking powder until the nuts are finely ground. Add the butter and process until the mixture has the consistency of coarse meal. Add the egg and process just until the dough forms a ball.

4. Divide the dough in half. With floured fingertips, pat each half evenly into one of two ungreased 9-inch square baking pans. Spread ½ cup of the jam evenly over the dough in each pan.

5. Scatter 2¼ cups of the streusel over each jam-coated square to cover the jam. Don't pat the streusel with your fingertips to pack it down.

6. Bake for 45 minutes, or until the streusel is light golden. Cool completely on a wire rack before cutting into squares. If desired, sprinkle lightly with confectioners' sugar or pipe thin lines of raspberry jam back and forth over the dessert's surface before cutting. Store at room temperature for 2 to 3 days or freeze for up to 2 weeks.

Variation

Chocolate Strata Bars: Coarsely grate 8 ounces semisweet chocolate. Sprinkle 4 ounces over each unbaked 9-inch square. Bake as directed. To decorate, pipe thin lines of melted white or dark chocolate back and forth over the baked surface.

YIELD: TWO 9-INCH PANS; 32 SQUARES

Indispensable Snack Cake

Whenever I visit Flo Braker, the most gifted baker I know, she has this cake on the kitchen counter, in a rectangular pan with its own sliding plastic cover. Flo says her family likes to snack on the cake day and night. I do too. She adapted the recipe from one that appeared over thirty years ago in *Sunset* magazine.

2¼ cups all-purpose flour

1½ teaspoons ground cinnamon

½ teaspoon salt

1 cup firmly packed light brown sugar

¾ cup vegetable oil

1 cup chopped walnuts or pecans

1 teaspoon baking powder

1 teaspoon baking soda

1 large egg

1 cup buttermilk

1. Preheat the oven to 350 degrees F, with a rack in the lower third. Grease and flour a 9-by-13-inch baking pan.

2. Sift the flour, ½ teaspoon of the cinnamon and the salt into a large bowl. Using a rubber spatula or whisk, briefly mix in the brown sugar to blend the ingredients. Stir in the oil, mixing well.

3. Remove ¾ cup of the flour-sugar mixture, loosely packed, and add to it the nuts in a small bowl. Add the remaining teaspoon of cinnamon. Using your fingertips, blend well. Set aside.

4. Stir the baking powder and baking soda into the remaining flour-sugar mixture. Blend in the egg and buttermilk until the mixture is smooth. Pour into the baking pan and sprinkle the nut mixture evenly over the batter.

5. Bake for about 35 minutes, or until a toothpick inserted in the center comes out clean. Serve cut into squares or oblong pieces.

YIELD: 12 SERVINGS

Fresh Ginger Cake

Another classic from Flo Braker, this is an abridged version of a popular recipe from *The Simple Art of Perfect Baking*. It's a light-textured, not-too-sweet cake perfumed with ginger and lemon. Serve with fruit or yogurt.

◆————————————————————————◆

1½ cups all-purpose flour
1   teaspoon baking soda
¼   teaspoon salt
½   cup (1 stick) unsalted butter, softened
½   cup firmly packed light brown sugar
¼   cup light molasses
¼   cup dark corn syrup
1   large egg
½   cup water
2   teaspoons grated lemon zest
2   teaspoons grated fresh ginger
    Confectioners' sugar, for dusting

◆————————————————————————◆

1. Preheat the oven to 350 degrees F, with a rack in the lower third. Grease and flour a 9-inch square baking pan.

2. Sift together the flour, baking soda and salt into a small bowl.

3. In a large bowl, with an electric mixer at medium speed, cream the butter and brown sugar until fluffy. Beat in the molasses, corn syrup and egg until the batter is creamy and smooth.

4. With the mixer on low speed, beat in the sifted dry ingredients alternately with the water, beginning and ending with the dry ingredients. Stir in the lemon zest and ginger.

5. Pour the batter into the pan and bake for about 35 minutes, or until the cake begins to contract from the sides of the pan. Cool 5 to 10 minutes in the pan; invert. Sprinkle very lightly with confectioners' sugar and serve bottom side up. Cut into 9 squares.

YIELD: NINE 2-INCH SQUARES

Banananut Coffee Cake

Peanut butter and banana produce a rich-tasting yet light-textured yellow cake, which has a faint note of coffee in the background. The cake is worth trying just to see how beautifully it goes with the luscious coffee–cream cheese frosting. The frosting recipe doubles easily. Try it spread on Raya's Chocolate Wafers (page 185) or on Best Banana Bread (page 232).

Cake
- 2½ cups cake flour
- 2½ teaspoons baking powder
- ½ teaspoon salt
- ½ cup brewed coffee
- 2 medium bananas, pureed (about ⅔ cup)
- ½ cup (1 stick) unsalted butter, softened
- ¼ cup smooth peanut butter
- ¾ cup firmly packed light brown sugar
- ¾ cup sugar
- 2 large eggs
- 2 teaspoons finely ground coffee
- 1 teaspoon pure vanilla extract

Frosting
- 2 tablespoons (¼ stick) butter, softened
- 2 tablespoons cream cheese, softened
- 1 cup confectioners' sugar, sifted, or more as needed
- 1 teaspoon finely ground coffee
- 1½ teaspoons instant coffee powder, dissolved in 1 tablespoon hot water

1. Preheat the oven to 350 degrees F, with a rack in the lower third. Butter and flour a 9-by-13-inch pan.

2. **Make the cake:** Sift together the cake flour, baking powder and salt into a small bowl; set aside.

3. Stir the brewed coffee into the pureed bananas in a small bowl; set aside.

4. In a large bowl, with an electric mixer on high speed, cream together the butter and peanut butter until smooth, about 2 minutes.

5. Add the brown sugar and cream on high for a minute. Add the sugar and cream on high for another minute.

6. Add the eggs, one at a time, beating well after each addition. Add the ground coffee and vanilla and beat on high until light and fluffy, about 3 minutes.

7. Add the flour mixture in 3 portions, alternating with the banana-coffee mixture, beating well on medium speed after each addition.

8. Pour the mixture into the pan. Bake for 45 to 50 minutes, or until the top is light gold and a toothpick inserted in the center comes out clean. Cool completely in the pan.

9. **Meanwhile, make the frosting:** Cream together the butter and cream cheese with an electric mixer on high speed until smooth, about 2 minutes.

10. Add the confectioners' sugar and ground coffee and cream together on high until smooth, about a minute.

11. Add the dissolved instant coffee and blend on medium speed until smooth; the consistency should be slightly thick and spreadable. If the frosting seems too thick, add a few drops of water; if it seems too thin, add more confectioners' sugar.

12. When the cake has thoroughly cooled, spread it with the frosting. Store, covered, in the refrigerator for up to 4 days.

YIELD: 24 PIECES

Gingered Applesauce Bread

This bread gets its texture from yogurt and applesauce and its zing from plenty of fresh ginger. Try cutting quarter-inch-thick slices and spreading them with apple butter. The moist bread will keep for several days, but after that, it is best toasted.

2	cups all-purpose flour
1	teaspoon baking soda
½	teaspoon baking powder
¼	teaspoon salt
¼	cup (½ stick) unsalted butter, softened
½	cup sugar
½	cup firmly packed dark brown sugar
2	large eggs, beaten
1	teaspoon pure vanilla extract
1¼	cups applesauce, preferably unsweetened
¼	cup plain yogurt
¼	cup grated fresh ginger
2	tablespoons pine nuts (optional)

1. Preheat the oven to 325 degrees F, with a rack in the middle. Grease and flour a 9-by-5-inch loaf pan.

2. Sift together the flour, baking soda, baking powder and salt into a small bowl; set aside.

3. In a large bowl, with an electric mixer on medium speed, cream together the butter and sugars until well blended. Add the eggs and vanilla and blend thoroughly on medium speed.

4. Add the applesauce, yogurt and ginger and mix thoroughly on medium speed.

5. Add the flour mixture and mix on low speed just until combined, about 30 seconds.

6. Pour the batter into the pan. Sprinkle the top with pine nuts, if desired. Bake for 1 hour and 20 minutes, or until a toothpick inserted in the center comes out clean. Cool on a rack and serve at room temperature. Refrigerate, covered, for up to 4 days or freeze, wrapped in plastic wrap, then in foil, for up to 4 months.

YIELD: ONE 9-BY-5-INCH LOAF

Mocha Pudding Cake

One of those desserts that delights both children and adults, this bakes into two chocolaty layers: one a cake and the other a pudding. Besides being fun to eat and easy to make, it contains very little fat.

---

1 cup all-purpose flour

1 tablespoon unsweetened cocoa powder

2 teaspoons baking powder

1 teaspoon instant coffee powder

½ teaspoon salt

¾ cup firmly packed light brown sugar plus ¼ cup for topping

2 tablespoons corn oil

1 teaspoon pure vanilla extract

½ cup brewed coffee plus 1 cup for topping

Vanilla ice cream, coffee ice cream or whipped cream, for topping

---

1. Preheat the oven to 350 degrees F, with a rack in the middle. Lightly grease four 1-cup soufflé dishes or ramekins.

2. Sift the flour, cocoa powder, baking powder, instant coffee and salt into a medium bowl.

3. Add the ¾ cup brown sugar, the oil, vanilla and ½ cup brewed coffee and mix thoroughly. Pour into the soufflé dishes.

4. Sprinkle 1 tablespoon of the brown sugar over the batter in each dish. Pour ¼ cup hot coffee over the sugar and batter in each dish. The mixture will look strange and lumpy, but it will transform into a wonderful dessert as it bakes.

5. Bake for 30 minutes, or until the cake layer begins to pull away from the sides of the pan. Serve warm, topped with vanilla ice cream, coffee ice cream or whipped cream. This cake is best served the day it is made, preferably soon after it is baked.

Variation

Bake the cake in an 8-inch square pan. Sprinkle on ¼ cup brown sugar, then pour on a cup of hot coffee. Bake for 45 minutes, or until the cake pulls away from the sides.

YIELD: 4 SERVINGS

Marvelous Mocha Cupcakes

Somewhere between a chocolate cake and a cheesecake, these cupcakes are wonderful. Even if you already have a good chocolate cupcake recipe, the deep coffee taste of these will make you change loyalty.

◆————————————————◆

Cupcakes
1½ cups all-purpose flour
½ cup sugar
½ cup firmly packed light brown sugar
¼ cup unsweetened cocoa powder
1 teaspoon baking soda
¼ teaspoon salt
1 cup brewed coffee
⅓ cup corn oil
1 tablespoon white vinegar
1 teaspoon pure vanilla extract

Topping
8 ounces cream cheese, softened
⅓ cup firmly packed light brown sugar
1 tablespoon sugar
2 teaspoons instant coffee powder, dissolved
in 1 teaspoon hot water
1 large egg
½ cup semisweet chocolate chips (optional)

◆————————————————◆

1. Preheat the oven to 350 degrees F, with a rack in the middle. Lightly grease 18 muffin cups.

2. **Make the cupcakes:** Sift together the flour, sugars, cocoa, baking soda and salt into a large bowl.

3. Make a well in the center of the dry ingredients. Add the brewed coffee, oil, vinegar and vanilla. With an electric mixer on medium speed, mix until smooth, about 2 minutes.

4. Divide the batter among the muffin cups. Set aside while preparing the topping.

5. **Make the topping:** With an electric mixer on medium speed, beat the cream cheese with the sugars until fluffy, about 2 minutes.

6. Scrape down the sides of the bowl, add the dissolved coffee and mix well on medium speed, about a minute.

7. Scrape down the sides and add the egg. Beat well on medium speed, about a minute; the mixture will be thin.

8. Spoon about a tablespoon of topping onto the center of each cupcake. If desired, sprinkle a few chocolate chips on the topping.

9. Bake for 25 minutes, or until a toothpick inserted in the center of the cupcakes comes out clean. The cream cheese topping will probably stick to the toothpick, but the chocolate cake should not.

10. Cool on a wire rack; store in a covered container in the refrigerator.

YIELD: 18 CUPCAKES

Vanilla Poppy Seed Cake

The flavors of this lovely vanilla-scented pound cake, subtler than the ubiquitous lemon version, ripen if the cake is held for a day before serving. It's nice topped with fresh blueberries or sliced strawberries.

- ½ cup poppy seeds
- ¾ cup milk
- ½ cup plain yogurt
- 2⅓ cups all-purpose flour
- 1 tablespoon baking powder
- ½ teaspoon baking soda
- ½ teaspoon salt
- 1 cup (2 sticks) unsalted butter, softened
- 1⅓ cups sugar
- 3 large eggs, separated
- 1 tablespoon pure vanilla extract

1. Preheat the oven to 350 degrees F, with a rack in the middle. Grease and flour a 10-inch tube pan.

2. In a small bowl, stir together the poppy seeds, milk and yogurt; set aside.

3. Sift together the flour, baking powder, baking soda and salt into a medium bowl; set aside.

4. In a large bowl, with an electric mixer on medium speed, cream together the butter and sugar until well blended, about 2 minutes. Add the egg yolks and vanilla and blend thoroughly, about a minute.

5. Add the flour mixture, alternating with the poppy seed mixture, starting and ending with the flour.

6. In a separate bowl, whisk the egg whites until stiff peaks form. Stir a spoonful of the whites into the poppy seed batter to lighten it, then gently stir in the remaining whites.

7. Pour the batter into the pan. Bake for 50 minutes, or until the cake is golden and a toothpick inserted in the center comes out clean.

8. Cool the cake on a wire rack completely before removing it from the pan. Serve sliced at room temperature. Refrigerate, covered, for up to 5 days or freeze for up to 4 months.

YIELD: ONE 10-INCH CAKE

Best Banana Bread

A no-nonsense, classic banana bread. Walnuts are the only extra. As always, extremely ripe bananas—black ones that look like they're ready for the compost heap—will produce the sweetest and best results. If you want to dress up this bread and add a bit of coffee flavor, make a half-batch of the frosting for Banananut Coffee Cake (page 222) and spread it lavishly over the top. Serve this bread when you need something homey in a hurry.

◆————————————————————————————◆

2   cups all-purpose flour
1   teaspoon baking soda
¼   teaspoon salt
½   cup (1 stick) unsalted butter, softened
½   cup sugar
½   cup firmly packed light brown sugar
2   large eggs, lightly beaten
1   teaspoon pure vanilla extract
3   very ripe bananas, pureed (about 1⅓ cups)
¾   cup chopped walnuts

◆————————————————————————————◆

1. Preheat the oven to 325 degrees F, with a rack in the middle. Grease and flour a 9-by-5-inch loaf pan.

2. Sift together the flour, baking soda and salt into a small bowl; set aside.

3. In a large bowl, with an electric mixer on medium speed, cream together the butter and sugars until well blended. Add the eggs and vanilla and blend thoroughly on medium speed.

4. Add the banana puree and mix on medium speed.

5. Add the sifted flour mixture and mix on low speed until combined, about 30 seconds. Mix in the walnuts, using a wooden spoon.

6. Pour the batter into the pan and bake for 1 hour and 25 minutes, or until a toothpick inserted in the middle comes out clean. The slow baking is

the key to achieving a moist, flavorful loaf. Cool in the pan for 15 minutes. Invert the cake onto a wire rack and turn right side up on the rack to finish cooling. You can eat this hot, but it's best to wait until the bread is at room temperature. Refrigerate, covered, for up to a week or freeze for up to 4 months.

YIELD: ONE 9-BY-5-INCH LOAF

Turkish Coffee Pear Bread

Yogurt and pear puree give this subtle fruit bread a surprisingly rich and creamy texture, and the coffee and cardamom flavors linger as a pleasing aftertaste. You may want to make two breads at the same time, since they freeze with exceptional success; wrap each loaf in plastic wrap and then foil before freezing.

◆———————————————————————————◆

2   cups all-purpose flour
1   teaspoon baking soda
¼   teaspoon salt
½   cup (1 stick) unsalted butter, softened
½   cup sugar
½   cup firmly packed light brown sugar
2   large eggs, lightly beaten
1   teaspoon pure vanilla extract
1¼ cups pear puree (about 4 very ripe pears, peeled,
    cored and pureed in a food processor)
¼   cup plain yogurt
4   teaspoons ground coffee (regular grind)
1   teaspoon ground cardamom

◆———————————————————————————◆

1. Preheat the oven to 325 degrees F, with a rack in the middle. Grease and flour a 9-by-5-inch loaf pan.

2. Sift together the flour, baking soda and salt into a small bowl; set aside.

3. In a large bowl, with an electric mixer on medium speed, cream together the butter and sugars until well blended, about 2 minutes. With the mixer running, add the eggs and vanilla and blend thoroughly, about a minute.

4. Add the pear puree and yogurt and mix thoroughly.

5. With the mixer off, sprinkle the ground coffee and cardamom over the batter. Pour the flour mixture over the top and, on low speed, mix it in just until combined.

6. Pour the batter into the pan and bake for 1 hour and 5 minutes, or until a toothpick inserted in the center comes out clean. Cool for 10 minutes in the pan. Invert the cake onto a wire rack and turn right side up on the rack to finish cooling. When completely cool, slice thinly.

YIELD: ONE 9-BY-5-INCH LOAF

Indian Rice Pudding

Coffee and finely chopped pistachios flavor this lovely cardamom-scented version of a nursery classic. It's wonderfully delicate and comforting too.

◆————————————————————————◆

6 cups milk
⅓ cup long-grain white rice, preferably basmati
¼ cup sugar
2 teaspoons ground coffee (regular grind)
8 cardamom pods
⅛ teaspoon freshly grated nutmeg
¼ teaspoon ground cardamom
1 teaspoon pure vanilla extract
2 tablespoons finely chopped pistachios

◆————————————————————————◆

1. Place the milk and rice in a heavy medium saucepan. Bring to a boil over high heat, lower the heat to a simmer and reduce by one-third, stirring occasionally, about an hour.

2. Stir in the sugar, ground coffee and cardamom pods. Continue to simmer over medium heat, stirring occasionally, and reduce by one-half, about 1 to 1½ hours; the mixture will be thick. Remove and discard the cardamom pods.

3. Stir in the nutmeg, ground cardamom and vanilla. Divide the pudding among 6 individual ½-cup serving dishes. Sprinkle each with a teaspoon of chopped pistachios. Alternatively, pour the mixture into a larger serving bowl and sprinkle the nuts on top. Refrigerate until firm and cool, at least 2 hours, before serving.

YIELD: 6 SERVINGS

Cappuccino Mousse

This strongly flavored, cloudlike classic mousse, from Flo Braker, has just enough gelatin to hold its shape but not too much to make it hard to spoon, as is so often true of chocolate mousse. It coolly and satisfyingly coats the tongue, like an extravagant espresso-bar concoction.

3   large eggs, separated
½   cup plus 2 tablespoons sugar
1   envelope unflavored gelatin
¼   cup plus 2 tablespoons Kahlúa or other coffee liqueur
⅔   cup strong brewed coffee or espresso
    Dash of salt
2   cups heavy cream

1. In a large bowl, with an electric mixer, beat the egg yolks on medium speed, adding the ½ cup sugar gradually until the mixture is pale yellow, about 2 minutes.

2. Sprinkle the gelatin over the ¼ cup coffee liqueur in a small bowl and let stand to soften, 5 to 10 minutes.

3. Heat the coffee in a small saucepan; do not let boil. Whisk the coffee into the yolk mixture. Return the mixture to the saucepan and cook over medium heat, whisking constantly, just until it simmers. Add the gelatin mixture and stir until thoroughly blended and dissolved. Set aside until cool and slightly thickened, stirring occasionally.

4. With an electric mixer, beat the egg whites with the salt until soft peaks form. Slowly beat in the remaining 2 tablespoons sugar.

5. Using the same beaters, whip the cream with the remaining 2 tablespoons coffee liqueur until soft but distinct peaks form.

6. Fold the meringue and the whipped cream alternately into the coffee mixture, beginning and ending with the cream. Spoon into dessert dishes, cover and chill thoroughly, at least 4 hours or overnight.

YIELD: 6 SERVINGS

Granita di Caffè

No dessert in all Italy is better than the shaved coffee ice at the Tazza d'Oro, the best espresso bar in Rome, near the Pantheon. All year, people stream out the many doors holding small plastic drink cups filled with the sweet, potent brown slush, topped with whipped cream. It isn't hard to make at home—you don't need an ice-cream maker—but it does require frequent trips to the freezer to get the right shaved-ice consistency.

- 2 cups water
- ½ cup sugar
- 1 cup freshly brewed coffee, brewed with 6 tablespoons (3 scoops) ground coffee
- 1 teaspoon pure vanilla extract
- ½ cup heavy cream, lightly whipped

---

1. In a small saucepan, heat a cup of the water with the sugar, stirring to dissolve the sugar; refrigerate until cold.

2. Combine the sugar syrup with the coffee, the remaining cup of cold water and the vanilla, and blend thoroughly. Pour into a freezer-safe container, such as a 9-by-13-inch metal pan.

3. Freeze, stirring and scraping the mixture with a rubber spatula at first and then with the tines of a fork every 30 to 40 minutes, until a grainy consistency is achieved and the mixture is completely frozen, about 3 to 4 hours.

4. Spoon the mixture into chilled glasses or bowls. Top each serving with a small dollop of softly whipped cream.

YIELD: 1 QUART

Toasted Hazelnut Ice Cream

Coffee and hazelnuts make perhaps the supreme ice-cream flavor. This classic ice cream from Flo Braker is rich, smooth and wonderful with cookies and coffee.

◆────────────────────────◆

    2   cups whole hazelnuts
    ¾   cup sugar
    1½ cups milk
    5   large egg yolks
    2   cups heavy cream
    1   tablespoon instant coffee powder
    1   teaspoon pure vanilla extract

◆────────────────────────◆

1. Preheat the oven to 350 degrees F. Spread the hazelnuts on a baking sheet. Toast for 15 to 20 minutes, until the smell permeates the air. To see if the nuts are toasted, cut one in half; it should be golden brown in the center. Remove from the oven and let cool slightly. To remove the skins, place the nuts on a tea towel, cover with another towel and rub; the skins will slip off.

2. Grind a cup of the nuts with ¼ cup of the sugar in a food processor until they are a powder. Chop the remaining cup of toasted nuts very coarsely; set aside.

3. Combine the milk and ground nuts in a large saucepan and set over medium-low heat. Meanwhile, beat the egg yolks in a large bowl, gradually adding the remaining ½ cup sugar. As the milk comes to the boil, strain a small amount into the yolks and mix well. Strain the remaining milk into the yolks, blending thoroughly.

4. Return the custard to the saucepan and bring just to the boil over medium heat. Add the cream, instant coffee and vanilla. Chill until cool, at least 4 hours.

5. Pour into an ice-cream maker and freeze according to the manufacturer's instructions. When the mixture has thickened but before it has frozen solid, fold in the coarsely chopped nuts. Freeze solid.

YIELD: ABOUT 1 QUART

White Coffee Truffles

Lisë Stern's fabulously smooth truffles—enrobed in chocolate, with their subtle filling of coffee-steeped cream, white chocolate and coffee liqueur filling—transcend normal truffles. What's more, these are easier than most to make.

◆━━━━━━━━━━━━━━━━━━━━━━━━━◆

Truffles
   3 tablespoons heavy cream
   1 teaspoon coffee beans (about 12)
   6 ounces white chocolate, finely chopped
   2 tablespoons (¼ stick) unsalted butter
   1 tablespoon Kahlúa or other coffee liqueur
      Confectioners' sugar, for dusting hands
Coating
   9 ounces semisweet or bittersweet chocolate,
      finely chopped
   2 teaspoons ground coffee (regular grind)

◆━━━━━━━━━━━━━━━━━━━━━━━━━◆

1. **Make the truffles:** *Microwave method:* Place the cream and coffee beans in a microwave-safe small bowl and microwave on high for a minute.

Stovetop method: Place the cream and coffee beans in a small saucepan and heat just until bubbles begin to form on the surface of the cream; remove from the heat.

2. Let stand for 30 minutes; remove the coffee beans and discard.

3. *Microwave method:* Combine the chopped white chocolate, cooled cream and butter in a microwave-safe small bowl. Heat on high for a minute. Remove from the microwave and stir. If the chocolate is still fairly solid, heat for another 30 seconds. Stir the mixture until smooth. If there still seem to be several unmelted pieces of chocolate, heat again for about 20 seconds, and then stir.

Stovetop method: Place the white chocolate, cooled cream and butter in the top of a double boiler. Bring the water in the bottom to a simmer. Stir the chocolate mixture occasionally, and as the chocolate begins to melt, stir more frequently until the mixture is smooth. Remove from the heat.

4. Add the coffee liqueur and stir until smooth.

5. Cover and refrigerate overnight. Alternatively, freeze for 2 hours. *(The mixture may be prepared in advance to this point and frozen for up to 3 months.)* When you are ready to form the truffles after a long freezing, place them in the refrigerator overnight; otherwise, the mixture will be too firm to form into balls.

6. Line a baking sheet with wax paper. Scoop the truffle mixture into rounded teaspoonfuls and drop the mounds onto the paper. Dust your hands with confectioners' sugar and roll the mounds into smooth balls. Place in the freezer for an hour or overnight.

7. **Make the coating:** *Microwave method:* Place the chopped chocolate in a microwave-safe medium glass bowl and heat on high for a minute. Stir until smooth. If the chocolate is still fairly solid, heat for another 30 seconds. Stir the mixture until smooth. If there still seem to be several unmelted pieces of chocolate, heat again for about 20 seconds, and then stir. Be careful, as the chocolate should not get too hot.

Stovetop method: Place two-thirds of the chopped chocolate in the top of a double boiler. Bring the water in the bottom to a simmer. Stir occasionally. As the chocolate begins to melt, stir in some pieces of the remaining chocolate. Do not let the melting chocolate get too hot. When most of the chocolate is melted but some lumps remain, turn off the heat and add the remaining chocolate; stir the mixture until smooth.

8. Stir in the ground coffee.

9. **Coat the truffles:** Remove the truffles from the freezer. Drop a truffle into the chocolate coating. Using 2 forks, roll it around to coat it thoroughly, then lift, letting the excess chocolate drip off. Return the truffle to the baking sheet. If desired, use a fork to drip a thin, decorative swirl of chocolate over the top. Repeat with the remaining truffles.

10. Let the truffles set in the freezer for about an hour. Refrigerate in an airtight container for up to 2 weeks or freeze for up to 6 months. Remove the truffles from the freezer about 20 minutes before serving.

YIELD: ABOUT 30 TRUFFLES

Chocolate-Hazelnut Truffles

Chocolate and dark-roasted hazelnuts are one of life's best combinations, and anyone who favors a buttery, impossibly rich truffle will love these. The praline takes some time to make but rewards the effort by keeping beautifully in the freezer for months. It also adds incomparable crunch to the hard bittersweet coating, which offers a complete contrast to the nearly liquid filling.

◆————————————————————————————————◆

Hazelnut Praline

1 cup whole hazelnuts

1 cup sugar

Truffles

8 ounces semisweet or bittersweet chocolate, finely chopped

½ cup (1 stick) unsalted butter, chilled and cut into 8 pieces

3 tablespoons brewed coffee

1 tablespoon Frangelico or other hazelnut liqueur

⅔ cup hazelnut praline

Unsweetened cocoa powder, for dusting hands

Coating

12 ounces semisweet or bittersweet chocolate, finely chopped

6 tablespoons hazelnut praline

◆————————————————————————————————◆

1. **Make the praline:** Preheat the oven to 350 degrees F. Spread the hazelnuts on a baking sheet. Toast for 15 to 20 minutes, or until the smell permeates the air. To see if the nuts are toasted, cut one in half; it should be golden brown in the center. Remove from the oven and let cool slightly. To remove the skins, place the nuts on a tea towel, cover with another towel and rub; the skins will slip off.

2. Lightly oil a sheet of foil; set aside.

3. In a small saucepan over medium heat, melt the sugar, stirring occasionally. It should start to melt after about 6 minutes. The sugar will be lumpy and granular, and look like a mistake. Persevere. Within the next few minutes, those lumps will melt into a smooth, amber-colored liquid. Lower the heat and

stir in the toasted hazelnuts, coating the nuts thoroughly. The mixture will be very sticky. Immediately scrape the mixture with a metal spoon (do not use a rubber spatula) onto the foil, spreading it out. Use a metal spoon dipped in water to flatten it. The praline will become brittle and difficult to pour as soon as you remove it from the heat, and you will not be able to scrape every last drop from the pan. Don't worry. (To clean the pan, soak it in hot, soapy water. The sugar will dissolve.)

4. Let the praline cool to room temperature, about 30 minutes. Break it into pieces and put it in a food processor. Pulse to chop as finely as possible into a lumpy powder. You should have 2 cups; the praline can keep indefinitely in an airtight container in the freezer.

5. **Make the truffles:** *Microwave method:* In a microwave-safe medium bowl, combine the chopped chocolate and butter. Heat on high for a minute. Stir until smooth. If the chocolate is still fairly solid, heat for another 30 seconds. Stir the mixture until smooth. If there still seem to be several unmelted pieces of chocolate, heat again for about 20 seconds, and then stir.

Stovetop method: Combine the chopped chocolate and butter in the top of a double boiler. Bring the water in the bottom to a simmer. Stir the chocolate mixture occasionally. As the chocolate begins to melt, stir more frequently until the mixture is smooth. Remove from the heat.

6. Add the coffee and hazelnut liqueur and stir until smooth.

7. Add the hazelnut praline and mix in thoroughly.

8. Cover and refrigerate overnight. Alternatively, freeze for 2 hours. *(The mixture may be prepared in advance to this point and frozen for 3 months.)* When you are ready to make the truffles after a long freezing, place them in the refrigerator overnight; otherwise, the mixture will be too firm to form into balls. Do not try warming it in the microwave—it will melt.

9. Line a baking sheet with wax paper. Scoop the truffle mixture into rounded teaspoonfuls and drop the mounds onto the paper. Dust your hands with cocoa and roll the mounds into smooth balls. Place in the freezer for at least an hour or overnight.

10. **Make the coating:** *Microwave method:* Place the chopped chocolate in a microwave-safe medium bowl and heat on high for a minute. Stir until smooth. If the chocolate is still fairly solid, heat for another 30 seconds. Stir the mixture until smooth. If there still seem to be several unmelted pieces of chocolate, heat again for about 20 seconds, and then stir. Be careful, as the chocolate should not get too hot or too liquid.

Stovetop method: Place two-thirds of the chopped chocolate in the top of a double boiler. Bring the water in the bottom to a simmer. Stir occasionally. As the chocolate begins to melt, stir in some pieces of the remaining chocolate. Do not let the melting chocolate get too hot. When most of the chocolate is melted but some lumps remain, turn off the heat and add the remaining chocolate; stir the mixture until smooth.

11. Stir in the hazelnut praline.

12. **Coat the truffles:** Remove them from the freezer. Drop a truffle into the chocolate coating. Using 2 forks, roll it around to coat it thoroughly, then lift, letting the excess chocolate drip off. Return to the baking sheet. If desired, use a fork to drip a thin, decorative swirl of chocolate over the top. Repeat with the remaining truffles.

13. Let the truffles set in the freezer for about an hour. Refrigerate in an airtight container for up to 2 weeks or freeze for up to 6 months. Remove from the freezer about 20 minutes before serving.

YIELD: ABOUT 30 TRUFFLES

Note: This praline is sensitive to weather. It prefers a cool and, especially, a dry climate. If the air is particularly humid, make the praline another day. This recipe makes more than is needed here, but praline is nice to have on hand and stores well in the freezer.

Mocha Truffles

The coffee-infused cream in the incredibly smooth filling of these truffles takes the sweet edge off the milk chocolate and adds a marvelously pronounced coffee taste. The casing of milk chocolate flecked with tiny bits of coffee sets off the filling without dominating it.

◆————————————————————————◆

Truffles
  1 teaspoon ground coffee (regular grind)
  ¼ cup heavy cream
  6 ounces milk chocolate, finely chopped
  2 tablespoons (¼ stick) unsalted butter
  1 tablespoon brewed coffee
  1 teaspoon pure vanilla extract
   Unsweetened cocoa powder, for dusting hands

Coating
  9 ounces milk chocolate, finely chopped
  2 teaspoons ground coffee (regular grind)
   Coffee beans (optional)

◆————————————————————————◆

1. **Make the truffles:** *Microwave method:* Add the ground coffee to the cream in a microwave-safe small bowl and microwave on high for 45 seconds.

Stovetop method: Place the ground coffee and the cream in a small saucepan and heat just until bubbles begin to form on the surface of the cream; remove from the heat.

2. Let stand for 30 minutes.

3. *Microwave method:* Combine the chopped milk chocolate and the butter in a microwave-safe medium bowl. Heat on high for 1 minute and 30 seconds. Remove from the microwave and stir. If the chocolate is still fairly solid, heat for another 30 seconds. Stir the mixture until smooth. If there still seem to be several unmelted pieces of chocolate, heat again for about 20 seconds, and then stir.

Stovetop method: Combine the milk chocolate and butter in the top of a double boiler. Bring the water in the bottom to a simmer. Stir the chocolate mixture occasionally. As the chocolate begins to melt, stir more frequently until the mixture is smooth. Remove from the heat.

4. Add the coffee-cream mixture, brewed coffee and vanilla and stir until smooth.

5. Cover and refrigerate overnight. Alternatively, freeze for 2 hours. *(The mixture may be prepared in advance to this point and frozen for up to 3 months.)* When you are ready to form the truffles after a long freezing, place in the refrigerator overnight; otherwise, the mixture will be too firm to form into balls.

6. Line a baking sheet with wax paper. Scoop the truffle mixture into rounded teaspoonfuls and drop the mounds onto the paper. Dust your hands with cocoa and roll the mounds into smooth balls. Place in the freezer for at least an hour or overnight.

7. **Make the coating:** *Microwave method:* Place the chopped chocolate in a microwave-safe medium bowl and heat on high for a minute. Stir until smooth. If the chocolate is still fairly solid, heat for another 30 seconds. Stir the mixture until smooth. If there still seem to be several unmelted pieces of chocolate, heat again for about 20 seconds, and then stir. Be careful, as the chocolate should not get too hot.

Stovetop method: Place two-thirds of the chopped chocolate in the top of a double boiler. Bring the water in the bottom to a simmer. Stir occasionally. As the chocolate begins to melt, stir in some pieces of the remaining chocolate. Do not let the melting chocolate get too hot. When most of the chocolate is melted but some lumps remain, turn off the heat and add the remaining chocolate; stir the mixture until smooth.

8. Stir in the ground coffee.

9. **Coat the truffles:** Remove the truffles from the freezer. Drop a truffle into the chocolate coating. Using 2 forks, roll it around to coat it thoroughly, then lift, letting the excess chocolate drip off. Return it to the baking sheet. If desired, top with a coffee bean. Repeat with the remaining truffles.

10. Let the truffles set in the freezer for about an hour. Refrigerate in an airtight container for up to 2 weeks or freeze for up to 6 months. Remove them from the freezer about 20 minutes before serving.

YIELD: ABOUT 30 TRUFFLES

Pistachio Truffles

When you just can't eat another bite of chocolate, try a spoonful of this filling—delicate white chocolate powerfully flavored with fresh pistachios. Then robe the candies with dark chocolate, and serve them with Mocha Truffles (page 245) for a luscious after-dinner array.

◆━━━━━━━━━━━━━━━━━━━◆

Truffles
- ⅓ cup shelled pistachios
  Corn oil, as needed
- 6 ounces white chocolate, finely chopped
- ¼ cup heavy cream
- 1 tablespoon unsalted butter
- ½ teaspoon pure vanilla extract
  Confectioners' sugar, for dusting hands

Coating
- 9 ounces semisweet or bittersweet chocolate, finely chopped
  About ⅓ cup pistachio pieces

◆━━━━━━━━━━━━━━━━━━━◆

1. **Make the truffles:** In a food processor, grind the pistachios until a paste forms. If the nuts are very dry, add the corn oil, ½ teaspoon at a time, with the machine running. The consistency of the paste should be like dry peanut butter; set aside.

2. *Microwave method:* Combine the chopped white chocolate, cream and butter in a microwave-safe medium bowl. Heat on high for a minute. Remove from the microwave and stir. If the chocolate is still fairly solid, heat for another 30 seconds. Stir the mixture until smooth. If there still seem to be several unmelted pieces of chocolate, heat again for about 20 seconds, and then stir.

Stovetop method: Combine the white chocolate, cream and butter in the top of a double boiler. Bring the water in the bottom to a simmer. Stir the chocolate mixture occasionally, and as the chocolate begins to melt, stir more frequently, until the mixture is smooth. Remove from the heat.

3. Add the vanilla and reserved pistachio paste and stir until smooth.

4. Cover and refrigerate overnight. Alternatively, freeze for 2 hours. *(The mixture may be prepared in advance to this point and frozen for*

up to 3 months.) When you are ready to form the truffles after a long freezing, place them in the refrigerator overnight; otherwise the mixture will be too firm to form into balls.

5. Line a baking sheet with wax paper. Scoop the truffle mixture into rounded teaspoonfuls and drop in mounds onto the paper. Dust your hands with confectioners' sugar and roll the mounds into smooth balls. Place in the freezer for at least an hour or overnight.

6. **Make the coating:** *Microwave method:* Place the chopped chocolate in a microwave-safe medium bowl and heat on high for a minute. Stir until smooth. If the chocolate is still fairly solid, heat for another 30 seconds. Stir the mixture until smooth. If there still seem to be several unmelted pieces of chocolate, heat again for about 20 seconds, and then stir. Be careful, as the chocolate should not get too hot.

Stovetop method: Place two-thirds of the chopped chocolate in the top of a double boiler. Bring the water in the bottom to a simmer. Stir occasionally. As the chocolate begins to melt, stir in some pieces of the remaining chocolate. Do not let the melting chocolate get too hot. When most of the chocolate is melted but some lumps remain, turn off the heat and add the remaining chocolate; stir the mixture until smooth.

7. **Coat the truffles:** Remove the truffles from the freezer. Drop a truffle into the chocolate coating. Using 2 forks, roll it around to coat it thoroughly, then lift, letting the excess chocolate drip off. Return to the baking sheet. Top with a piece of pistachio. Repeat with the remaining truffles.

8. Let the truffles set in the freezer for about an hour. Refrigerate in an airtight container for up to 2 weeks or freeze for up to 6 months. Remove from the freezer about 20 minutes before serving.

Yield: About 30 truffles

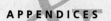

Sources

My watchcry is: buy local. If you have a store near you that roasts beans carefully and sells coffee-making equipment, do your best to keep it in business—assuming, of course, that you like what it sells. One of the most heartening trends of the past decade has been the flowering of neighborhood roasters, and it would be sad to see them eclipsed by specialty chains, just as regional wholesale roasters were long ago undersold and driven out of business by big national brands. Fresh is always better.

You can get fresh beans by mail, of course—sometimes fresher than your local store provides, especially if it receives infrequent shipments of beans and leaves them in bins exposed to light and air. Geography doesn't matter that much in mail order. A company that is closer to you will often charge less for shipping, and its beans might arrive a day sooner; but considering that supermarkets keep beans out for weeks, it doesn't make much difference. The point is to find a place, if you don't have one nearby, that will explain to you which beans are especially good at the time you call—and to settle on a supplier whose beans and roast style please you.

This guide is by no means comprehensive. I haven't been to every city in the country, and each time I visit a new town, I'm happily surprised by the new variety of shops selling beans and equipment and doing a terrific job of it. Instead, I point out a few places that I know from experience to be reliable and to be equipped to handle mail orders.

I've roughly divided the companies by those that sell equipment, those that sell beans and those that sell both. If a company that roasts beans is listed under Equipment, it's because the equipment it sells is hard to find anywhere else in the country. You can assume that each company (except for individual manufacturers) sells a wide range of products; specific pieces of equipment or kinds of coffee are listed in the entries below because they are mentioned in the text.

Beans

Allegro Coffee Company

12799 Claude Court
Building B, Dock 4
Thornton, CO 80241
(303) 444-4844/(800) 277-1107
Fax: (800) 530-3993
www.allegrocoffee.com

Allegro sells numerous organic coffees, including Guatemala La Magnolia, and single-origin coffees, such as Kenya Grand Cru, Costa Rican Dota Tarrazu and Sulawesi Toraja.

Batdorf & Bronson Coffee Roasters

200 Market Street NE
Olympia, WA 98501
(800) 955-5282/(360) 754-5282
Fax: (360) 754-5283
www.batdorf.com
E-mail: javatalk@batdorf.com

The independent and dedicated roaster Batdorf & Bronson offers a number of organic and single-origin coffees, as well as several of its own blends. Customers who choose the "Carefree" subscription program receive two seasonal coffees by mail each month.

Caffé D'arte

719 South Myrtle Street
Seattle, WA 98108
(800) 999-5334/(206) 762-4381
Fax: (206) 763-4665
www.caffedarte.com
E-mail: info@caffedarte.com

The artisan roaster Mauro Cipolla sells from Seattle more than a dozen hand-crafted coffees for drip and espresso

makers. Two of Caffé D'arte's blends, Velletri and Fabriano, are prepared in special wood-fired roasting machines from Cipolla's native Italy. These are especially highly regarded by espresso addicts.

Castle & Company

2118 Wilshire Boulevard
Suite 634
Santa Monica, CA 90403
(310) 479-5999/Fax: (310) 312-1762

Castle & Company, a champion of beans raised and processed with special care, sells a full selection of green coffee beans to roasters.

Coffee Bean International, Inc.

2181 NW Nicolai Street
Portland, OR 97210
(503) 227-4490/(800) 877-0474
Fax: (503) 225-9604
www.coffeebeanintl.com

CBI sells a full line of specialty coffees—including certified organic and Fair Trade coffees—and teas to specialty-food stores and coffee shops.

Distant Lands Coffee Roasters

13081 State Highway 64 West
Tyler, TX 75704-9493
(888) 262-5282/Fax: (903) 593-2699
www.dlcoffee.com
E-mail: sales@dlcoffee.com

Distant Lands Coffee Roasters sells an array of whole-bean coffees, including beans from La Minita in Costa Rica, and other estate-grown coffees from Kenya, Ethiopia, Jamaica and Colombia, as well as a selection of blends and flavored coffees.

Espresso Vivace Roasteria

901 East Denny Way
Seattle, WA 98122
(206) 860-5869
Fax: (206) 860-1567
www.espressovivace.com
E-mail: vivace@speakeasy.net

Master barista David Schomer is a
nexus for espresso fanatics across the
country. He sells by mail the two coffee
blends served at his famed Seattle
café Espresso Vivace, along with his
own instructional books and videos on
making espresso.

J. Martinez & Company

3934-3936 Green Industrial Way
Atlanta, GA 30341-1914
(800) 642-5282/(404) 231-5465
Fax: (404) 233-6528
www.martinezfinecoffees.com

J. Martinez & Company specializes in
single-estate Jamaican coffees—especially Jamaica Blue Mountain, of which it
is among the only reliable sources in the
country. John Martinez had been a coffee grower in Jamaica before moving to
Atlanta and starting the company in
1988. Martinez has built and maintained
close relations with growers of premium
coffees from around the world and buys
and roasts the highest grades. The company serves the luxury market, as its
packaging, which is especially beautiful,
shows.

Knutsen Coffees, Ltd.

San Francisco, CA
(800) 231-7764/Fax: (415) 922-1045

Erna Knutsen, a wholesaler long revered in the specialty-coffee trade, sells
a full array of specialty green beans to
wholesalers and roasters. If you are having trouble finding a particular bean,
chances are good that her office will
know where to buy it.

Schapira's Coffee & Tea Co.

P.O. Box 327, Factory Lane
Pine Plains, NY 12567-0327
(518) 398-7100/Fax: (518) 398-7137
E-mail: schapira@taconic.net

Joel Schapira (now retired) and his
family have been leaders in bringing
quality arabica coffee to East Coast customers, and the company bearing their
name carries on the tradition, with carefully selected and just-roasted beans.

Equipment

Alessi USA Inc.

155 Spring Street, 4th Floor
New York, NY 10012
(212) 431-1310
Fax: (212) 431-1390
www.alessi.com
E-mail: alessi@alessiusa.com

Alessi, the Italian tableware designer,
sells two versions of the plunger pot,
one designed by Michael Graves and one
by Aldo Rossi. Other products include
teapots, cream pitchers and sugar bowls.

Bodum

413-415 West 14th Street
New York, NY 10014
(212) 367-9125/(800) 232-6386
Fax: (212) 367-9128
www.bodum.com

Bodum, the Danish manufacturer,
makes a whole line of coffee equipment,
including plunger pots in many sizes

(Bodum bought the most famous producer of them, the French Melior) and vacuum pots—including the sleekly designed, electrified Santos models, which finally provide a convenient alternative to electric drip machines, using the finest brewing method for non-espresso coffee.

Boyd Coffee Company

19730 NE Sandy Boulevard
Portland, OR 97230
(503) 666-4545/Fax: (503) 669-2223
www.boyds.com
E-mail: info@boyds.com
Boyd Coffee, one of the West Coast's principal roasters of beans, sells top-notch brewing equipment, including the Dutch-made Technivorm home electric brewer, which is hard to find.

Braun

(800) 272-8611
www.braun.com
Braun, the large German appliance manufacturer, sells a range of reliable electric drip coffee makers, propeller grinders and burr mills.

Brewing Market

2525 Arapahoe Avenue
Boulder, CO 80302
(303) 444-4858/(800) 628-9170
Fax: (303) 447-9579
Brewing Market, also a roaster, sells two sizes of the very hard to find English Cona glass vacuum brewer.

The Brita Products Company

P.O. Box 24305
Oakland, CA 94623-9981

(800) 542-7482 (for filters and replacement parts)
(800) 242-7482 (for store locations)
Brita sells a well-distributed line of water filtration pitchers for home use.

DeLonghi America, Inc.

P.O. Box 3900
Peoria, IL 61612
(800) 322-3848
www.delonghiusa.com
E-mail: delonghiconsumer@
    speedymail.com
DeLonghi, the Italian appliance manufacturer, makes more than fifteen different espresso makers, including pump machines, steam machines and combination drip and espresso/cappuccino makers.

Espresso Specialists, Inc.

4544 Leary Way NW
Seattle, WA 98107
(800) 367-0235/(206) 784-9563
Fax: (206) 784-9582
www.esi-online.com
E-mail: esi@esi-online.com
Espresso Specialists is an importer and distributor of top-of-the-line commercial Italian espresso machines, which a national network of dealers installs in espresso bars.

Espresso Supply

1123 NW 51st Street
Seattle, WA 98107
(206) 782-6670/(800) 782-6671
Fax: (206) 789-8221
www.espressosupply.com
E-mail: info@espressosupply.com
Espresso Supply carries more than 150 different espresso accessories that are

often unavailable from stores that sell espresso machines, including knock boxes, tampers, steaming pitchers, thermometers and cleaning products, including Puro Caff powder.

Fante's
1006 South 9th Street
Philadelphia, PA 19147
(800) 443-2683/Fax: (215) 922-5723
www.fantes.com
E-mail: mail@fantes.com
This long-established kitchen-equipment and gourmet store in Philadelphia's Italian neighborhood, which sells many kinds of beans, is noteworthy for its wide choice of equipment, including stainless-steel napoletana brewers, Chemex brewers and also plastic funnels for the overnight cold-water brewing method.

1st-Line Equipment
www.1st-line.com
E-mail: sales@1st-line.com
1st-Line Equipment sells a variety of hard-to-find espresso machines to home and commercial users, as well as a full selection of grinders, coffees and accessories.

Krups
(800) 526-5377
www.krups.com
Krups markets a full selection of propeller grinders and coffee and espresso machines, including machines compatible with the E.S.E. pod system and the Perfect Froth attachment, which enhances milk-steaming wands on home espresso machines.

Sivetz Coffee, Inc.
349 SW 4th Street
Corvallis, OR 97333
(541) 753-9713/Fax: (541) 757-7644
www.sivetzcoffee.com
E-mail: info@sivetzcoffee.com
Michael Sivetz, an inventor, manufacturer and curmudgeon in the American coffee business, offers by mail a variety of green coffees and roasters to professionals and dedicated amateurs. He also sells reprints of his authoritative books on coffee technology.

Sur La Table
84 Pine Street
Seattle, WA 98101
(800) 243-0852/Fax: (206) 448-2245
www.surlatable.com
Sur La Table carries a wide range of coffee-making items, including stovetop espresso makers in stainless steel, pots for Middle Eastern coffee, stainless-steel coffee measures and thermal carafes.

Williams-Sonoma
P.O. Box 379900
Las Vegas, NV 89137-9900
(800) 541-2233/Fax: (702) 363-2541
www.williams-sonoma.com
Williams-Sonoma sells packaged coffee from Illy and electric brewers from Krups, as well as an assortment of grinders, brewers and espresso makers.

Beans & Equipment

Caribou Coffee Company, Inc.
615 North 3rd Street
Minneapolis, MN 55401
(888) 227-4268

www.cariboucoffee.com

With about 200 stores in eight states, Caribou Coffee sells a wide range of whole-bean and ground coffees from New Guinea, Colombia, Ethiopia, Kenya and Indonesia.

Gillies Coffee Company

150 19th Street
Brooklyn, NY 11232
(718) 499-7766/(800) 344-5526
Fax: (718) 499-7771
www.gilliescoffee.com
E-mail: info@gilliescoffee.com

Gillies Coffee, "the oldest coffee merchant in America," offers a wide array of choice whole beans and custom blends, including Jamaica Blue Mountain, along with brewing and grinding equipment.

Green Mountain Coffee Roasters

33 Coffee Lane
Waterbury, VT 05676
(800) 223-6768/Fax: (802) 244-1395
www.gmcr.com
E-mail: CustomerCare@gmcr.com

Green Mountain Coffee Roasters, long known for its environmentally friendly practices and products, such as its oxygen-bleached paper filters, offers a wide range of beans, including Jamaica Blue Mountain, La Minita Tarrazu and Yemen Mocha Sanani, in addition to a full selection of brewing and grinding equipment.

illycaffè North America, Inc.

200 Clearbrook Road
Elmsford, NY 10504
(800) 872-4559/(914) 784-0500
www.illyusa.com
E-mail: info@illyusa.com

Illy, the revered Italian roaster, sells a large selection of its coffees roasted and ground for espresso, espresso-making equipment and a sought-after series of artist-designed espresso cups.

Lavazza Premium Coffees Corp.

(800) 466-3287/Fax: (212) 725-9475
www.lavazzausa.com
E-mail: info@lavazzausa.com

Lavazza, Italy's largest coffee roaster, sells a wide variety of espresso blends and also coffee-making equipment, including stainless-steel moka stovetop espresso makers.

Peet's Coffee and Tea

P.O. Box 12509
Berkeley, CA 94712-3509
(800) 999-2132/Fax: (510) 594-2180
www.peets.com

Peet's, long a California cult and for thirty-five years the inspiration for specialty-coffee roasters across the country, offers a full range of fresh-roasted coffees, and espresso and coffee-brewing machines.

Porto Rico

201 Bleecker Street
New York, NY 10012
(212) 477-5421/(800) 453-5908
Fax: (212) 979-2303
www.portorico.com

Porto Rico sells stainless-steel moka stovetop espresso pots, Pavoni and Saeco espresso machines and also 140 different coffees.

Starbucks Coffee Company

P.O. Box 34067
Seattle, WA 98124-1510
(800) 782-7282/Fax: (800) 782-7286
www.starbucks.com

Starbucks, which has become synonymous in America with espresso drinks and efficient service, sells a full selection of beans, brewers, grinders and accoutrements. Under its Barista brand it sells two espresso machines, the Barista and the Barista Athena, which both have the invaluable adjustable filter holder that increases pressure before brewing.

Sweet Maria's

www.sweetmarias.com
E-mail: info@sweetmarias.com

Primarily a source for green coffee beans and home roasting machines, the Internet retailer Sweet Maria's also sells a full selection of brewing equipment and gives access to an extensive database of coffee-cupping reviews.

Thanksgiving Coffee Company

P.O. Box 1918
Fort Bragg, CA 95437
(800) 648-6491/Fax: (707) 964-0351
www.thanksgivingcoffee.com

Thanksgiving, known for its environmental consciousness, sells both retail and wholesale organic coffee, Swiss Water Process decaffeinated coffees and shade-grown coffees. Much of its coffee is certified as part of the Fair Trade program (see TransFair USA, page 258).

Whole Latte Love

www.wholelattelove.com
E-mail: sales@wholelattelove.com

An online retailer, Whole Latte Love sells a wide variety of espresso makers, grinders, home roasters, brewing accessories and coffee blends. Especially useful are the site's numerous product reviews, demonstration videos and

head-to-head comparisons of different machines.

Zabar's

2245 Broadway
New York, NY 10024
(800) 697-6301/(212) 496-1234
Fax: (212) 580-4477
www.zabars.com
E-mail: info@zabars.com

Besides its own coffees, Zabar's offers a large selection of burr and propeller coffee grinders and home espresso pump machines.

Organizations

Coffee Kids

1305 Luisa Street, Suite C
Santa Fe, NM 87505
(505) 820-1443/(800) 334-9099
Fax: (505) 820-7565
www.coffeekids.org
E-mail: info@coffeekids.org

Coffee Kids is an international nonprofit organization that works to improve living conditions for children and families in coffee-growing communities worldwide.

Equal Exchange

251 Revere Street
Canton, MA 02021
(781) 830-0303/Fax: (781) 830-0282
www.equalexchange.com
E-mail: info@equalexchange.com

Equal Exchange, which in 1991 became the first American retailer to sell Fair Trade coffee (see TransFair USA, page 258, for a brief summary of Fair Trade requirements), today buys coffee from farmers' cooperatives in ten countries and claims to be the largest U.S. coffee merchant (it is a for-profit company, alone among the groups listed here) whose entire line of products meets Fair Trade standards.

Global Exchange

2017 Mission Street #303
San Francisco, CA 94110
(415) 225-7296/Fax: (415) 255-7498
www.globalexchange.org
E-mail: info@globalexchange.org

Through a network of campus and community activists, this international social-justice organization lobbies American roasters to sell Fair Trade coffee.

Grounds for Health

286 College Street
Burlington, VT 05401
(800) 375-3398/Fax: (802) 865-3364
www.groundsforhealth.org
E-mail: groundsforhealth@coffee-ent.com

Co-founded by Dan Cox, of Coffee Enterprises, and Jon Wettstein, of Green Mountain Coffee Roasters, Grounds for Health aims to improve health-care facilities in coffee-growing communities in Mexico and Central America.

International Coffee Organization

22 Berners Street
London, W1T 3DD, England
+44 (0)20 7580 8591
Fax: +44 (0)20 7580 6129
info@ico.org

Since 1963 the ICO, based in London, has been the United Nations of coffee, bringing together more than sixty coffee-producing and coffee-consuming countries and providing a forum for disputes between countries and between the representatives of farmers, governments and private companies. Through its International Coffee Agreement, a frequently renegotiated treaty, the ICO helped regulate the world supply and price of coffee, greatly aiding farmers in producing countries. Like the UN, the ICO has had its moments of disunity: disagreements over quotas and price regulation led producing and consuming countries to withdraw from the agreement, beginning a period of instability in the price of coffee. Today the ICO is revitalizing itself, launching new initiatives to promote sustainable agriculture and to maintain its longtime role as the world's foremost collector and distributor of authoritative information on coffee.

Oxfam

26 West Street
Boston, MA 02111-1206
(800) 776-9326/(617) 482-1211
Fax: (617) 728-2594
www.oxfamamerica.org
E-mail: info@oxfamamerica.org

Oxfam's Coffee Rescue Plan seeks to stabilize the coffee market by advocating equitable trade practices to governments and coffee companies and improving international coffee quality standards; as a way to raise the prices of good coffee, Oxfam suggests in its plan the destruction of some of the surplus low-quality coffee that gluts the world market.

Specialty Coffee Association of America Resource Center

One World Trade Center, Suite 1200
Long Beach, CA 90831
(562) 624-4100/Fax: (562) 624-4101
www.scaa.org
E-mail: coffee@scaa.org

The Specialty Coffee Association of America, which tracks an industry that has in the past twenty years seen explosive growth, sells its own reprints of William Ukers's classic book *All About Coffee*, as well as a wide selection of educational and training materials.

TechnoServe

49 Day Street
Norwalk, CT 06854
(800) 999-6757/Fax: (203) 838-6717
www.tns.org
E-mail: technoserve@tns.org

A nonprofit group that promotes entrepreneurship in developing countries, TechnoServe helps coffee farmers in Africa and Latin America gain better access to markets and raise the prices farmers are paid by improving the quality of the beans they grow.

TransFair USA

1611 Telegraph Avenue, Suite 900
Oakland, CA 94612
(510) 663-5260/Fax: (510) 663-5264
www.transfairusa.org
E-mail: transfair@transfairusa.org

To receive the Fair Trade label, importers and roasters must agree to buy directly from farmers and growing cooperatives, extend credit to producers against future sales, promote environmentally sustainable agricultural practices and pay farmers a minimum price per pound. TransFair USA is the independent monitoring organization responsible for certifying Fair Trade coffees in the United States.

Internet Resources

Alt.coffee Newsgroup

groups.google.com (search for "alt.coffee")

A lively electronic message board frequented by veterans and amateurs alike, alt.coffee is a good place to share tips or seek advice about buying and brewing.

CoffeeGeek

www.coffeegeek.com
E-mail: info@coffeegeek.com

The online community CoffeeGeek is home to more than a thousand reviews of different brewers, grinders and accessories, written by both experts and home users. The site also features commentary from a group of regular columnists and electronic discussion forums.

Coffee Kid

www.coffeekid.com
E-mail: questions@coffeekid.com

Mark Prince, one of CoffeeGeek's founders, also maintains his own website, which is a good resource for espresso novices.

Coffee Review

www.coffeereview.com
E-mail: editor@coffeereview.com

A panel of expert cuppers, led by the food writer Kenneth Davids—himself a national authority and guru—rates coffees on a 100-point scale for acidity, aroma, body and flavor.

Glossary

Acidity—Not a defect, acidity is one of the reasons the best high-grown arabica coffee beans fetch the highest prices. As a roast gets going, flavorful acids form, giving coffee life and sparkle. The lighter the roast, the more the acids are highlighted; very dark roasts destroy most acids. Not to be confused with bitterness.

Adenosine—One of the chemicals, or neurotransmitters, the body makes to control neural activity, adenosine triggers a series of slowing effects in the body. Researchers think caffeine acts as an adenosine impostor, locking into special receptors on brain cells and fooling the body into thinking that adenosine is circulating when it is not. Caffeine thus speeds you up by not slowing you down.

Aged coffees—Green coffee beans that have been stored in the climate, typically hot and humid, in which they were grown, for a year or two or even three before being shipped. Similar to monsooning, which takes less time, aging beans is expensive, because stocks are tied up. Aged coffee has a soft roundness many connoisseurs seek, especially for blends.

Air-quenching—The cooling of roasted beans with blown air rather than with sprayed water (see water-quenching).

Arabica—One of the two main coffee species. *Coffea arabica* is named for its original popularizers, the Arabs, who brought it from its native East Africa to the Arabian Peninsula in the fifteenth century. All the delicate, prized flavors possible in coffee are found in arabica and not robusta, the other main species, although not every arabica is fine. Arabica beans, which produce the best flavors when grown at high altitudes in semitropical climates near the equator, naturally contain about half the caffeine (an average of 1.1 percent) of robusta beans (which have an average of 2.2 percent).

Barista—The Italian name for the master of the espresso machine.

Bitterness—A catchall term used to express displeasure with the taste of coffee. Coffee is naturally bitter, but should not be unpleasantly so. When the natural bitterness of caffeine is removed in decaffeinated coffee, the flavor balance is thrown off. Bitterness becomes unpleasant when coffee is underroasted, highlighting its chlorogenic acid, or when it is overheated on a burner—America's chief coffee crime.

Blend—A mixture of beans from different parts of the world and sometimes at different roasts, as opposed to a straight coffee, which is coffee from one region. A roaster usually has secret recipes for signature house blends.

Body—A tasting term to describe the weight of coffee on the palate. Paper-filtered coffee is typically light in body; coffee brewed through a metal screen, as in a plunger pot and in all espresso, typically has a more viscous and a sometimes syrupy body. Beans themselves have different degrees of body depending on where they are grown and on their species; arabica beans have lower body than robusta beans.

Boiler—The small tank in an espresso machine used to heat water and steam milk. Room-temperature water for espresso is drawn by a pump directly from the reservoir through a copper pipe that travels through the boiler before delivering the hot water to the filter holder.

Bourbon—A hallowed variety of the arabica species, named for the French island colony off Africa (today Réunion) where it once grew. Bourbon, the basis of the Latin American trade for hundreds of years, is an impractical choice for a farmer today, because its yield is one-third to one-half that of many newer arabica varieties. Because connoisseurs prize its flavors and are willing to pay more for Bourbon beans, growers in such countries as Guatemala and Nicaragua are replanting Bourbon trees where they were torn out or abandoned.

Brick pack—Coffee beans or, more frequently, ground coffee that has, in effect, been shrink-wrapped in thick plastic bags. Brick packs, which save both the price of metal for cans and storage space, were developed in Germany in the 1950s but only decades later came into wide use in the United States. They are no better than a can for preserving flavor, because both storage methods require that the coffee first be degassed.

Burr mill—A grinder whose two shredding discs, or burrs, are grooved and can be adjusted to be closer or farther apart, depending on how fine or coarse a grind is necessary. Although they are more expensive than propeller grinders, burr mills work much more slowly and are even noisier. Nonetheless, they offer precision and consistency that make all the difference in everyday brewing.

Café au lait—A French breakfast drink made up of about one-third strong brewed coffee, as in coffee from a café filtre or napoletana pot or the stovetop moka brewer, and two-thirds scalded or steamed milk. Virtually identical to the Italian family version of a caffè latte.

Café filtre—The metal flip-drip pot, more commonly called by its Italian name, *napoletana,* used in French households. The Italians like to claim credit for it, but in fact the French invented the device in the early nineteenth century.

Caffè americano—In Italy, usually a thin drink made with instant coffee. In America, an espresso lengthened with plain hot water after brewing (not by brewing for a longer time), so that the body is about the same as that of a filter-brewed coffee. A good way to spread out the taste of espresso over a longer sipping time without adding cups of milk.

Caffè latte—In Italy (where it is spelled *caffelatte*), this is a family drink made in the morning with coffee brewed in the napoletana or moka and milk scalded on the stove, in proportions of roughly 1 part coffee to 3 parts milk. Italian espresso bars use genuine espresso and sometimes add more steamed milk, but not as much as is used in the United States. Also, Italians don't add foamed milk, as Americans usually do. The drink served as a "latte" in American coffee bars is really a giant-sized cappuccino.

Caffè macchiato—An espresso "stained" with about two tablespoons of foamed milk.

Caffeine—The chief mood-altering substance in coffee, with an average of 1.1 percent in arabica and 2.2 percent in robusta beans, the two main coffee species. When extracted, as in the decaffeination process, caffeine is a pure white crystal, bitter to taste. Caffeine is the world's most widely used psychoactive drug, appearing naturally in tea leaves and, in very small quantities, in cocoa beans.

Caffeine intoxication—Psychiatric diagnosis indicated by five or more of the following signs that occur during or shortly after caffeine is consumed (generally over 250 milligrams, the amount in two or three cups of coffee): restlessness, nervousness, excitement, flushed face, diuresis (increased urination), gastrointestinal disturbance, muscle twitching, rambling flow of thought and speech, tachycardia or cardiac arrhythmia, periods of inexhaustibility, and psychomotor agitation. The diagnosis is made only if these symptoms cause clinically significant distress or impairment in social or occupational functioning.

Caffeine withdrawal—Not yet an official diagnosis, but a syndrome currently under research for possible inclusion in psychiatric manuals. Its symptoms

include headache, sleepiness or drowsiness, impaired concentration, difficulty working, depression, anxiety, irritability, nausea and vomiting, and muscle aches or stiffness.

Cappuccino—An espresso-based drink classically made with one-third espresso, one-third steamed milk and one-third foamed milk. The king of Italian espresso drinks.

Caramelization—Beans are naturally high in carbohydrates, which must be heated to develop toasty, sweet flavors. Caramelized sugars give body and mouthfeel to a darker roast: the darker the bean, the higher the degree of caramelization. When caramelization is taken too far, coffee tastes burnt.

Cezve—More commonly called an ibrik, this is the correct term for the long-handled brass or copper pot, tinned on the interior, that slopes inward at the top and is used to make Middle Eastern coffee.

Cherry—Coffee beans are the seeds of a berry, called a cherry for the shape and for the deep crimson color of the fully ripe fruit. The even, ovoid shape resembles a plump holly berry or cranberry.

Chlorogenic acid—One of the principal acids in green coffee beans, unpleasantly astringent by itself. As the roast progresses, much of the chlorogenic acid disappears and other, flavorful acids form, more than making up for its loss.

Cinnamon roast—The lightest roast commercially available, with no oil on the surface. Large manufacturers often incorporate very light roasted coffee into their blends, because roasting for a short time both saves money and adds bulk. A cinnamon roast rarely appears in specialty shops, though, because it is so high in chlorogenic acid and low in body and flavor.

City roast—A roasting term controversial for its imprecision but in wide use. Today a city roast is barely darker than a cinnamon roast. "Full-city" is used for a medium roast, more or less dark cinnamon in color and with no oil on the surface; this is the fullest development of a bean before oils appear. The next stage is usually called a Vienna roast.

Clean cup—A term professional tasters use to indicate a brewed coffee that is free, or virtually free, of taste defects. A clean coffee is not the same as a great coffee, but it will bring the grower or broker a higher price.

Colloids—Suspended particles of coffee solids that are too large to dissolve fully but small enough to pass through a metal filter (but not through a paper filter). Often called brew colloids, these give coffee its texture and mouthfeel. They are also an important component of crema.

Cowboy coffee—Ground coffee steeped in hot water and then strained to separate grounds from brew. Legend has it that the separation method often called for a clean sock into which the ground coffee was spooned before being immersed in water. (Also called hobo, campfire or open-pot coffee.)

Crema—A golden foam made up of oil and colloids, which floats atop the surface of a perfectly brewed cup of espresso.

Achieving crema depends on a number of factors, including kind of coffee used, its freshness and the degree of pressure used in brewing; achieving it is tricky when not using a professional espresso machine.

Cupcake filter—Flat-bottomed coffee filter with ridged sides, familiar from restaurant filter-drip machines and household Mr. Coffee brewers. Many experts find this shape superior to the familiar wedge.

Cupping—The process by which professional tasters evaluate a sample of beans. Roasted and ground coffee is steeped in hot water, like tea, and the liquid is tasted both warm and as it cools.

Decaffeination—The removal of caffeine from green coffee beans by any of a number of processes, including methylene chloride, water process, Swiss Water Process, and supercritical carbon dioxide. The actual amount of caffeine remaining in decaffeinated beans varies, more because of the care that different companies take than because of the process itself.

Defects—A range of problems that professional tasters may find in samples of beans from importers and brokers. Among the most common are ferment and underripeness. Less common defects include an iodinelike flavor called "Rio-y," a "hidey" flavor from beans washed with tainted water or shipped too close to tanned leather hides, and a rubbery flavor from beans grown near rubber trees.

Degas—When beans are roasted, they produce up to three times their volume in carbon dioxide gas, which must be released before they are packaged in a sealed container, such as a can or brick pack, to avoid bursting. Unfortunately, while the beans release carbon dioxide, they also absorb oxygen, which is why some people dismiss what comes out of a brick pack or can as pre-staled coffee. Standard paper bags, for short-term storage, or valve-lock bags, for long-term storage, avoid this problem.

Dirty cup—Coffee that shows any of several taste defects.

Diuretic—Anything that makes you empty your bladder. Caffeine is a diuretic and will require you to drink other fluids in order to compensate for the ones it draws out.

Drip coffee—The most common home-brewing method, also called brewed coffee, by which hot but not boiling water drips through ground coffee at the force of gravity (espresso requires much greater force), preferably into a thermal carafe.

Drip pot—Most commonly used to refer to multi-compartmented dime-store metal coffeepots. Except for the fact that almost all American drip pots are made of aluminum, which interacts with coffee, they are a fine way to make coffee.

Dry process—Also called unwashed or natural process, this is sun-drying of coffee cherries to ferment the sticky mucilage, or pulp, that encases the beans, or seeds. In dry-processing, fermentation takes place outdoors, either on raised racks or on the ground; the dry husk is then broken and the mucilage scraped off. Generally considered infe-

rior to the more expensive washed process. Still, many discerning tasters look for and enjoy the flavor of dry-processed beans, which they say have an earthy power that washed coffees lack.

Dwell time—The amount of time it takes a home espresso machine to heat water in the boiler from the temperature required for brewing to that required for steaming—as much as fifty degrees higher. The wait can be long. It is eliminated in thermal-block machines.

Electric drip—The standard coffee brewer in American kitchens, ever since the launch of Mr. Coffee in the early 1970s. Electrically heated water drips through a paper or metal filter into a carafe, usually glass. To avoid burning brewed coffee, always transfer it immediately to a thermal carafe. Or throw it out after fifteen minutes.

Espresso—A method of brewing coffee by forcing hot water at high pressure through finely ground coffee, producing a syrupy texture and a powerful, sweet taste. Refers to the method of brewing, not to the kind of bean or color of the roast. The required pressure can be produced only in a pump or piston machine.

Ethyl acetate—A chemical used to decaffeinate coffee by a "direct" process, meaning that the solvent comes into direct contact with the green beans before being heated and evaporated. Used by some large companies (Procter & Gamble, which produces Folgers, for example) as an alternative to methylene chloride, and sometimes called naturally decaffeinated because ethyl acetate occurs in small quantities in fruits like bananas and apples. Considered inferior both to methylene chloride, because it is less specific to caffeine and so carries away flavor as well, and to the improved Swiss Water Process.

Extraction rate—The amount of soluble solids that pass from coffee beans to brewed coffee and give it body and flavor. The shorter the brewing time, the finer the grind must be, so that the extraction will be quick and thorough. If the brewing time is long, the grind should be coarse, to avoid overextracting undesirable substances.

Filter holder—The part of a professional or home espresso machine that holds the ground coffee, this consists of a small metal filter that fits into a big metal handle. The filter holder (also called a portafilter) latches into the group of the espresso machine, which channels hot water through the ground coffee. Espresso flows out a spout, or two spouts, at the bottom of the filter holder.

Fines—The powdery dust of finely ground coffee. The only brewing method that officially requires beans ground this fine is Middle Eastern coffee. But because so much grinding equipment is imprecise, ground coffee usually contains some ratio of fines—too much of which clogs filters.

Flip-drip pot—Identical to a napoletana or café filtre pot.

Fluid-bed roaster—A type of hot-air roaster, first developed in the 1920s, which keeps beans aloft in a "fluid" stream of hot air; the process itself is very dry. Manufacturers of the machines say they produce beans with a cleaner flavor and greater volume, because the beans puff before they lose much water. Many in the specialty trade maintain that these machines roast beans too fast and sacrifice full flavor.

Foamed milk—Milk both heated and aerated with a steam wand. Foam builds at the top of the milk pitcher during the end of the steaming process. The ideal consistency of foamed milk is of very lightly whipped cream that just holds its shape.

French press—*See* Plunger pot.

French roast—The vaguest of the controversial names for roasts, this means different things on different coasts of the United States—either very dark or so dark as to be almost black, with a gloss of oil on the surface. The French don't roast this dark, and many connoisseurs think nobody else should either.

Gold filter—Metal filter plated with gold for durability. Made in sizes to fit most coffee makers, wedge or cupcake, these filters allow more colloids into the brew and thus produce a thicker-textured and more satisfying coffee.

Green beans—The seeds of a coffee fruit, removed from the cherry (the whole fruit) and either dry-processed or washed to remove them from the sticky mucilage in which they were suspended. Green beans are seldom a deep green (some Indonesian beans are jade green), but they are usually pale—between a light green hay color and a dull beige straw color.

Ground coffee—Roasted coffee beans that have been put through some kind of grinder. Grounds that have already been used for brewing are called spent grounds or coffee grounds.

Group—The area of a professional or home espresso machine—usually a thick metal circle with grooves, like a European light socket—into which the filter holder, filled with ground coffee, is latched.

Harrar—A growing region of Ethiopia known for its fruity, winy, dry-processed beans.

Italian roast—Like French roast, a vague term usually referring to an extremely dark roast, covered with a gloss of oil. Also like French roast, this has nothing to do with the country for which it is named, which usually roasts beans much lighter.

Java—One of the main islands of Indonesia, which the Dutch colonized in the eighteenth century and made a center of coffee production. So successful were they that "Java" has remained slang for coffee.

Knock box—A useful accoutrement to a home espresso machine, a knock box is a square metal box the size of a largish ashtray with a rubber-coated bar mounted at the top. Used as a receptacle for spent grounds.

Meta-analysis or Meta-survey—Retrospective assessment of many thematically related studies, even if they were conducted over a number of years and in many parts of the world by unconnected laboratories. Public-health officials often rely on meta-analyses as the basis for their advice, for example, whether people should avoid or reduce caffeine or coffee consumption.

Metal filter—Perforated screen, often a gold filter, that allows water to pass through ground coffee to make brewed coffee. Unlike paper filters, metal filters allow colloids to pass through them, resulting in a thicker-textured and, to some, a more satisfying brew.

Methylene chloride—The most efficient chemical solvent to decaffeinate coffee in a "direct" process, meaning that the solvent comes into contact with the green beans (the water process is indirect). To date, this produces the best-tasting decaf. In 1985, the FDA declared the risk of methylene chloride in decaffeination to be so low "as to be essentially non-existent." The amount of methylene chloride left in brewed coffee is parts per billion—less than in the air of many cities.

Middle Eastern coffee—A brew made by boiling ground coffee several times, very briefly, in a long-handled brass or copper pot, called a cezve or ibrik. The froth at the top—the sign of an expert maker—is distributed equally among the guests as a gesture of respect. This is a sweeter and lighter coffee than its technique or its reputation suggest. Different countries, notably Turkey and Greece, have their own variations of this method.

Milds—Coffee-business term for all arabica beans that don't come from Brazil. Not a flavor description: Brazilian arabicas, though important in the world coffee trade, are so dull that they play almost no part in specialty coffee.

Mocha—The original name of the port on the Arabian Peninsula (*Al Mukha* in Arabic), through which the first cultivated coffee, from eastern Africa and the country now called Yemen, was shipped. In Europe, "mocha" became synonymous with coffee, and when chocolate arrived from the New World, it was thought to be similar in taste. Today, beans from Yemen—the only ones that can truly be called Mocha beans—are extremely rare. But the word "mocha" lives on, to describe anything with the combination of coffee and chocolate and also as part of the first and still most famous coffee blend, Mocha-Java.

Mocha-Java—Classically, a combination of half Yemen and half Java beans, blended to balance the wildness and acidity of a Yemen-style coffee with the heavy body and earthy richness of Indonesian coffee. Blends called Mocha-Java at a supermarket or coffee shop seldom contain a single bean of either true Mocha or Java coffees. Beans from Yemen are scarce and expensive (thus the more common ratio of one-third Yemen to two-thirds Java), and beans from Java are often considered overpriced for their quality, so roasters use just about anything they feel like in the blend.

Moka—A common name and a brand name for the stovetop brewer typically used in every Italian household, with a cinched waist and faceted sides, popularized in the 1930s by its first large-scale manufacturer, Bialetti. In a moka, water boils in a closed chamber with enough headroom to allow steam to collect. The pressure from the steam forces the hot water to escape from the chamber and pass through the ground coffee. What comes out is drip coffee with a push. Although the moka does not achieve the pressure necessary for true espresso, it produces coffee that makes a fine base for milk drinks like cappuccinos and lattes.

Monsooning—The process of aging a coffee in order to simulate the temperature and humidity fluctuations to which beans in the eighteenth and nineteenth centuries were subjected on their voyages from the Arabian Peninsula or Africa to and from Europe; customers found the mellow flavors pleasing. "Aged coffee" is usually aged many more months; "monsooning" is now used to denote beans from India that have been held in a hot, humid place for a few months.

Napoletana—Metal flip-drip pot beloved in Italian households, frequently called a macchinetta in Italian-American shops. The device has two cylindrical pots, one atop the other, one with a spout, and between them a separate compartment for ground coffee. After water boils in the lower chamber, the pot is flipped over and the water drips through the ground coffee into the part with a spout. Produces a strong brew with much of the body people admire in plunger-pot coffee.

Natural process—*See* Dry process.

Paper filter—Absorbent paper barrier used in brewing filtered coffee. Today, oxygen-bleached filters are the safest bet for those who care both about the environment and how coffee tastes. Many people admire the purity of paper-filtered coffee; others prefer the thicker texture of coffee brewed through a metal filter.

Parchment—A hard, beige jacket around a coffee bean like a thin pistachio shell that remains after the bean is washed or dry-processed. Beans can be stored for many months in their parchment without flavor changes. Before shipping, the parchment is rubbed off in a polishing machine.

Percolation—The filtering of liquid through a perforated metal or even a ceramic screen. The device we call the percolator is properly a "pumping percolator," because it recycles boiling water through ground coffee, producing a bitter, sour brew. Water should pass through ground coffee just once—something that happens during true percolation.

Piston machine—Forerunner of today's pump machine, this uses a hydraulically powered piston to produce the pressure necessary to make true espresso. The big lever on the front of a professional piston machine opens a powerful spring, allowing greater control over the "pull" of the espresso—named for the motion made when pulling down the lever—than does the pushbutton on a pump machine. The Pavoni, a manual home piston machine, lacks the spring.

Plunger pot—Also called a French press or Melior, after the longtime French manufacturer of it. Coffee grounds steep in water, like tea leaves, for six minutes. Then a finely perforated metal screen is pressed down through the liquid to separate the grounds from the brewed coffee. The brew is the thickest-textured of any except stovetop and professional espresso.

Polishing—Removing the parchment and much of the silverskin of a coffee bean by friction, for cosmetic purposes, before it is shipped.

Propeller grinder—Small pedestal-style hand-held electric coffee grinder with a spinning blade. These are inexpensive and unobtrusive, but they hold only small quantities of coffee beans and are extremely imprecise. Burr mills are far more consistent in producing a specific grind size.

Pump machine—Espresso brewer that, using a small electric pump, produces high pressure to force hot but not boiling water through finely ground coffee, producing true espresso. All high-quality home espresso machines (ones that cost at least $100) include a pump. Professional machines use pumps or pistons.

Pyrolysis—The chemical changes that occur during roasting when the interior of the bean produces heat of its own, breaking down the bean's raw components and forming hundreds of new aromatic volatile compounds.

Reservoir—The chamber at the back of an espresso machine that holds fresh water. Always make sure there is fresh cool water in the reservoir before you turn on a home espresso machine. (Professional machines are plumbed.)

Roaster—Literally, the machine in which beans are roasted. In the coffee trade, the term generally means the person operating the machine. A roaster at a small or medium-sized coffee business frequently also selects and blends beans. In this case, he or she can be called a roastmaster.

Roasting—The heating process that releases all the potential flavors locked in green beans. In the specialty-coffee trade, this is most commonly done by spinning the beans in a drum heated by a gas flame.

Robusta—One of the two main coffee species, *Coffea canephora* is commonly called robusta for the name under which it was first promoted, which referred to its hardiness. It is frowned on in the specialty-coffee trade for its paper-bag flavor. Robusta grows very well at sea level, unlike the other main species, *Coffea arabica,* which grows best at high altitudes. Native to West rather than East Africa, robusta was first cultivated widely only a hundred years ago, for its low cost. Big commercial packagers around the world rely on robusta to fill out their blends, and many Italians rely on robusta's large body to give espresso its necessary syrupy texture.

Silverskin—Papery chaff that adheres to the green bean, usually visible in patches or a webbed pattern on its surface. Most silverskin dries into something resembling onionskin, and much of it wafts off during roasting. Silverskin also winds all the way inside the bean and is often visible as beige flecks in ground coffee.

Single-estate coffee—Beans grown on one farm in one country or coffee-producing region.

Soluble solids—All the substances that can be dissolved from coffee beans, only some of which should end up in brewed coffee. Roasted coffee beans contain about 30 percent soluble solids, and most experts put the ideal extraction rate at 18 to 22 percent.

Spent grounds—Used ground coffee. Good for compost. Not good to reuse in anything you plan to drink.

Steam machine—An espresso brewer that functions by steam pressure alone rather than by pressure from a pump or piston. The pressure forces hot water—not steam—to pass through the ground coffee. All stovetop espresso machines, such as the moka, work by simple steam pressure, as do inexpensive electric espresso and cappuccino machines (under $100), even if they are rigged out to look like household pump machines. The far greater pressure of pump or piston is necessary for true espresso.

Steam wand—Tube attached to home and professional espresso machines, which delivers steam through pinprick holes in a nozzle at the end; used chiefly to make steamed and foamed milk.

Steamed milk—Milk that has been heated by the injection of steam. Its volume is unchanged, unlike that of foamed milk.

Straight coffee—The beans of one region or country, not part of a blend.

Supercritical carbon dioxide—Decaffeination process in which carbon dioxide, under great pressure, becomes a fluid between the liquid and gaseous states and passes through steamed unroasted coffee beans to remove caffeine without removing other solids. When the pressure is eased, the fluid vaporizes and dissipates, leaving no trace.

Swiss Water Process—A decaffeination method similar to the water process except that only charcoal filters are used to remove caffeine—never chemicals, as are sometimes used in the water process.

Tamper—Small tool, typically plastic, used to press down and polish the surface of ground coffee loaded into the metal filter of a filter holder for an espresso machine. A tamper should be slightly narrower than the filter and have a flat bottom. The pressure should always be gentle.

Thermal block—A way of heating water in home electric espresso pump machines by spiraling hot water through a metal-alloy block, like a radiator, instead of heating it in a boiler. Thermal-block machines are quieter than other pump machines and take up less counter space, but frequently they do not produce the pressure necessary for excellent espresso.

Thermal carafe—Insulated container popularly known as a thermos. A carafe is the best way to store brewed coffee; keeping coffee on a burner overheats it, producing a sour, bitter brew. Even in a thermal carafe with a very tight seal, however, the holding time for brewed coffee is barely three-quarters of an hour before flavor deteriorates.

Unwashed process—*See* Dry process.

Vacuum-packed—Refers to the process of using a vacuum to remove air from coffee cans in order to preserve freshness. Vacuum packaging actually removes only 90 percent of the air in cans, leaving enough oxygen to stale the coffee, albeit slowly. A worse problem for freshness is the time it takes coffee to degas before being packaged: while carbon dioxide leaves, oxygen enters, in effect pre-staling the coffee. Also, in packaged ground coffee, the vacuum process sucks up aromatics, removing flavor.

Valve-lock bags—Packaging that incorporates a one-way valve to let out the carbon dioxide naturally released by roasted beans without letting in air. This allows freshly roasted beans to be packaged much sooner after roasting than do other packaging materials, which require beans to be first degassed.

Vienna roast—One of several controversial names for roasts. Usually refers to the stage at which the beans are chocolate brown, handsomely speckled with dark brown. Also traditionally describes a blend of beans taken to several different roast degrees.

Washed process—Coffee beans that have been fermented and put through channels of running water to remove the seed, or bean, from the sticky mucilage of the coffee cherry. This process results in a far cleaner cup than the much less expensive, and more common, dry process.

Water process—"Indirect" decaffeination process in which all the soluble solids, including caffeine, are removed from green coffee beans by soaking them in water. The water solution is then drained off and caffeine extracted. The thick liquid containing the soluble solids is returned to the waiting beans for reabsorption. The water process can involve chemicals at the point when the liquid is decaffeinated; very small amounts of chemical residues can be returned to the beans. The Swiss Water Process uses charcoal filters, not chemicals, to separate out caffeine.

Water-quenching—The cooling of roasted beans with sprayed water. When done properly, the water evaporates; when done improperly, the process adds water weight to beans.

Bibliography

Alessi. *Tea and Coffee Piazza.* 5th ed. Crusinallo: Shakespeare & Company, 1986.

American Psychiatric Association. *Diagnostic and Statistical Manual of Mental Disorders.* 4th ed. Washington, D.C.: American Psychiatric Association, 1994.

Bar Giornale. *Un Caffè Per Favore: L'Espresso Al Bar In Italia.* Milan: Pubbli-stampa Edizioni, 1989.

Bersten, Ian. *Coffee Floats, Tea Sinks.* Sydney: Helian Books, 1993.

Bramah, Edward, and Joan Bramah. *Coffee Makers: 300 Years of Art & Design.* London: Quiller Press, 1989.

Calvert, Catherine, and Jane Stacey. *Coffee: The Essential Guide to the Essential Bean.* New York: Hearst Books, 1994.

Camporesi, Piero. *Il Brodo Indiano.* Milan: Garzanti Editore, 1990.

Capodici, Salvatore, and Carlo Invernizzi. *Conoscere Il Caffè.* Milan: Ed. Eusebianum, 1983.

Castle, Timothy James. *The Perfect Cup.* Cambridge, Massachusetts: Perseus Publishing, 1991.

Cei, Lia Pierotti. *Il Caffè: Storie e ricette.* Milan: Mursia Editore, 1982.

Cheney, Ralph Holt. *Coffee: A Monograph of the Economic Species of the Genus Coffea L.* New York: New York University Press, 1925.

Clark, R. J., and R. Macrae, eds. Barking, Essex: Elsevier Applied Science
  Coffee: Volume 1: Chemistry
  Coffee: Volume 2: Technology
  Coffee: Volume 3: Physiology
  Coffee: Volume 4: Agronomy
  Coffee: Volume 5: Related Beverages
  Coffee: Volume 6: Commercial and Technico-Legal Aspects

Dalisi, Riccardo. *La Caffettiera e Pulcinella.* Milan: Officina Alessi, 1987.

Davids, Kenneth. *Coffee: A Guide to Buying, Brewing, & Enjoying.* 5th ed. New York: St. Martin's Press, 2001.

———. *Espresso: Ultimate Coffee.* 2nd ed. New York: St. Martin's Press, 2001.

———. *Home Coffee Roasting: Romance & Revival.* New York: St. Martin's Press, 1996.

DeMers, John. *The Community Kitchens Complete Guide to Gourmet Coffee.* New York: Simon & Schuster, 1986.

Desmet-Grégoire, Hélène. *Les Objets du Café.* Paris: Presses du C.N.R.S., 1989.

Ferré, Felipe. *Il Caffè.* Milan: Silvana Editoriale, 1988.

Fumagalli, Ambrogio. *Macchine da Caffè/Coffee Makers.* English translation by Johannes Henry Neuteboom. Milan: BE-MA Editrice, 1990.

Garattini, Silvio, ed. *Caffeine, Coffee, and Health.* New York: Raven Press, 1993.

Gordon, Jean. *Coffee.* Woodstock, Vermont: Gramercy Publishing Company, 1963.

Hattox, Ralph S. *Coffee and Coffeehouses: The Origins of a Social Beverage in the Medieval Near East.* Seattle and London: University of Washington Press, 1985.

Heise, Ulla. *Coffee and Coffee Houses.* West Chester, Pennsylvania: Schiffer Publishing, 1987.

Illy, Andrea Viiani Rinantonio. *Espresso Coffee: The Chemistry of Quality.* London and San Diego: Academic Press, 1995.

Illy, Francesco, and Ricardo Illy. *The Book of Coffee: A Gourmet's Guide.* Milan: Mondadori, 1989. 1st American ed., New York: Abbeville Press, 1992.

Jacob, Heinrich Eduard. *Coffee, The Epic of a Commodity.* Translated by Eden and Cedar Paul. New York: Viking Press, 1935.

Jacobs Suchard Museum. *Das Wiener Cafè.* Zurich, 1989.

Janssen, Phillip. *Espresso Seattle Style Quick Reference Guide.* Seattle: Peanut Butter Publishing, 1993.

Jobin, Philippe. *Les Cafés Produits dans le Monde.* English translation by Natalie Wagner-Marzocca, with technical collaboration by Jacques Combet. Le Havre, France: P. Jobin et Cie., 1982. (Available by mail from S.A.A.A., Boîte Postale 145, 76050 Le Havre, Cedex, France. Tel.: 35-19-35-00.)

Jobin, Philippe, and Bernard Van Leckwyck. *Le Café: Le Goût de la Vie.* Paris: Editions Nathan, 1988.

Jurich, Nick. *Espresso from Bean to Cup.* Seattle: Missing Link Press, 1991.

Knox, Kevin, and Julie Sheldon Huffaker. *Coffee Basics: A Quick and Easy Guide.* New York: John Wiley & Sons, Inc., 1996.

Kolpas, Norman. *The Coffee Lover's Companion.* New York: Quick Fox, 1977.

———. *A Cup of Coffee.* New York: Grove Press, 1993.

La Marzocco. *Coffee-Machines for Use in Bars.* Florence, 1991.

Laurence, Janet. *A Little Coffee Cookbook.* San Francisco: Chronicle Books, 1992.

Lavazza. *Guida al Caffè.* Milan: Centro Luigi Lavazza, 1991.

Lingle, Ted R. *The Coffee Cupper's Handbook.* Washington, D.C.: Coffee Development Group, 1986.

———. *The Basics of Cupping Coffee.* Long Beach, California: Specialty Coffee Association of America, 1988.

Mariano, Bernard. *Crema.* Chicago: Trendex International, Inc., 1991.

Mariano, Bernard N., and Jill West. *The Espresso Encyclopedia.* Chicago: Trendex International, Inc., 1994.

McCoy, Elin, and John Frederick Walker. *Coffee and Tea.* 3rd ed. San Francisco: G. S. Haly, 1991.

McHugh, Edna. *The Coffee Cookbook.* Los Angeles: Price, Stern, Sloan Publishers, 1973.

Michel, Sergio. *The Art and Science of Espresso.* Trieste: Illy Caffè, 1994.

Norman, Jill. *Coffee.* New York: Bantam Books, 1992.

Odello, Luigi. *Caffè E Cappuccini: Come Soddisfare I Palati Più Rari Ed Esigenti.* Sommacampagna, Italy: Demetra, 1993.

Olsen, Dave. *A Passion for Coffee.* Menlo Park, California: Sunset Books, 1994.

Pendergrast, Mark. *Uncommon Grounds: The History of Coffee and How It Transformed Our World.* New York: Basic Books, 2000.

Perry, Sara. *The Complete Coffee Book.* San Francisco: Chronicle Books, 1991.

Roden, Claudia. *Coffee.* London: Pavillion Books, 1987. 1st American ed., New York: Random House, 1994.

Rolnick, Harry. *The Complete Book of Coffee.* Hong Kong: Melitta, 1982.

Rothfos, Bernhard. *Coffee Production.* English translation by Sabine Buken. 2nd ed. Hamburg: Gordian-Max-Rieck GmbH, 1985.

———. *Coffee Consumption.* Hamburg: Gordian-Max-Rieck GmbH, 1986.

Schapira, Joel, David Schapira and Karl Schapira. *The Book of Coffee and Tea.* 2nd ed. New York: St. Martin's Press, 1982.

Schiaffino, Mariarosa. *Le Ore del Caffè.* 2nd ed. Milan: Idealibri, 1984.

Schomer, David C. *Espresso Coffee: Professional Techniques.* Seattle: Peanut Butter Publishing, 1996.

Sivetz, Michael. *Coffee Processing Technology.* Westport, Connecticut: Avi Publishers, 1963.

———. *Coffee Origin and Use.* Self-published, 1977.

———. *Coffee Technology.* Westport, Connecticut: Avi Publishers, 1979. (Reprints of the three Michael Sivetz books, which are out of print, are available from Sivetz Coffee; see page 254.)

Spiller, Gene A. *The Methylxanthine Beverages and Foods: Chemistry, Consumption, and Health Effects.* New York: Alan R. Liss, Inc., 1984.

Sturdivant, Shea, and Steve Terracin. *Espresso!* Freedom, California: The Crossing Press, 1991.

Svicarovich, John, Stephen Winter and Jeff Ferguson. *The Coffee Book: A Connoisseur's Guide to Gourmet Coffee.* Englewood Cliffs, New Jersey: Prentice-Hall, 1976.

Tekulsky, Mathew. *Making Your Own Gourmet Coffee Drinks.* New York: Crown Publishers, 1993.

Ukers, William H. *All About Coffee.* 2nd ed., 1935. Long Beach, California: Specialty Coffee Association of America, 1993. (Facsimile reprint available from the Specialty Coffee Association; see page 258.)

von Hünersdorff, Richard. *Coffee: A Bibliography.* London: Hünersdorff, 2002.

Weinberg, Bennett Alan, and Bonnie K. Bealer. *The World of Caffeine.* New York: Routledge, 2001.

Wrigley, Gordon. *Coffee.* Harlow, Essex: Longman Scientific & Technical; New York: John Wiley & Sons, Inc., 1988.

General Index

Recipe Index

About the Author

Called "a dean among food writers in America" by the *San Francisco Examiner,* Corby Kummer is one of the country's most respected journalists. He has served as a senior editor of *The Atlantic Monthly* since 1981. In addition to writing regularly about food and travel for the magazine, he is responsible for editing many articles on politics and the arts. His 1990 series on coffee was nominated for a National Magazine Award. Kummer also writes for many other magazines, including the *New York Times Magazine, Boston, Gourmet* and *Bon Appétit.* He wrote the authoritative chapters on coffee and tea for the new edition of *Joy of Cooking.* He is the author of *The Pleasure of Slow Food: Celebrating Authentic Traditions, Flavors, and Recipes.*